The Clinical Diagnosis and Treatment for New Coronavirus Pneumonia

Fanjun Cheng • Yu Zhang
Editors

The Clinical Diagnosis and Treatment for New Coronavirus Pneumonia

PMPH
PEOPLE'S MEDICAL PUBLISHING HOUSE

Springer

Editors
Fanjun Cheng
Department of Internal Medicine
Union Hospital, Tongji Medical College of Huazhong University of Science and Technology
Wuhan
China

Yu Zhang
Department of Pharmacy
Union Hospital, Tongji Medical College of Huazhong University of Science and Technology
Wuhan
China

ISBN 978-981-15-5977-8 ISBN 978-981-15-5975-4 (eBook)
https://doi.org/10.1007/978-981-15-5975-4

Jointly published with People's Medical Publishing House, PR of China

This Springer imprint is published by the registered company Springer Nature Singapore Pte Ltd.
The registered company address is: 152 Beach Road, #21-01/04 Gateway East, Singapore 189721, Singapore

Preface

Wuhan, China, as the initial place for the outbreak of COVID-19, not only had the cases from the earliest time, but also one of the largest infected populations until now. At the beginning of this outbreak, the Chinese government gathered professional and experienced medical staff to support Wuhan nationally. Meanwhile, 46 hospitals were designated as specialized institutions for the COVID-19 patients. 16 mobile cabin hospitals were newly built to accept patients with mild or moderate symptoms, and 7 large general hospitals were designated for severe or critical cases.

The West Campus of Wuhan Union Hospital, affiliated with the Tongji Medical College of HUST, is the one of the medical centers which accepted the largest number of severe and critical patients during the epidemic. By 24:00 on March 20, 2020, a total of 1671 severe and critical COVID-19 patients were treated in the hospital. The number of patients who had been successfully cured and discharged from the hospital was 1069, and 147 patients died. At that time, there were still 401 severe and critical cases in-house.

By making full use of its comprehensive medical power combined with specialists' skills of the 18 medical teams supporting Hubei, the West Campus of Wuhan Union Hospital has achieved better therapeutic accomplishments through comprehensive and personalized treatment, combined with early rehabilitation and psychological intervention. COVID-19 patients may also have medical conditions such as pregnancy, parturition, and urgent surgical conditions. It is still a great challenge to deal with these situations appropriately while ensuring the cure of COVID-19 and the protection of the medical staff.

Based on the "Guidelines for the diagnosis and treatment of COVID-19" issued by the National Health Commission of PRC, this manual is prepared not only by referring to the research results of modern medicine and combining with the specific circumstances of patients, but also by considering the allocation of medical resources. The content of this manual includes medical administration under emergent circumstances, prevention and control of nosocomial infection, clinical experience on the diagnosis and therapy, radiographic inspection, laboratory diagnosis, inhibition of inflammatory cytokine storm, convalescent plasma therapy, TCM, etc. It is a collection of wisdom and practice of medical institutions at the highest level in China to cope with COVID-19. We believe the publication of this manual will benefit the countries which are currently dealing with COVID-19.

One Earth, One Family. During the pandemic, nobody can step aside. China's practice experience and outcome to combat COVID-19 will enable the rest of the world not to start from scratch but continue in China's footsteps and fight the pandemic more effectively. As the Chinese government is exporting anti-epidemic personnel and materials to the world, we collected valuable information and experience from Wuhan Union Hospital by 18 medical troops from 12 provinces nationally during the past 2 months. We wish it is helpful for the prevention and control of COVID-19 in other countries.

Wuhan, China
March 26, 2020

Fanjun Cheng
Yu Zhang

Acknowledgments

The book is written and finally published with the support of all parties, including the full cooperation of the medical management personnel from the West Campus of Wuhan Union Hospital, and the unremitting efforts of medical and nursing staff from 21 national medical teams mainly composed of those from Union Hospital. These medical professionals organized and wrote the contents of this book in their spare time after high-intensity work shifts treating COVID-19 patients. Our special thanks also go to Mr. Anbang Cheng, a volunteer who has just graduated from the Faculty of Agricultural, Life and Environmental Sciences in the University of Alberta, and temporarily suspends his study at the Faculty of Environmental Science in the University of Melbourne due to the epidemic. In addition to providing volunteer service in the hospital logistics, he also made basic and great efforts for the English translation and organization of the book after the volunteer service. He is also the volunteer with the longest period of service in the West Campus of Wuhan Union Hospital for the COVID-19 prevention and control in Wuhan.

We would like to thank Dr. Zhongbo Hu from Case Western Reserve University, USA, and Mu Hu, Solon High School Student, Solon, OH, USA, for their timely and free services in finalizing the English manuscript, and the People's Medical Publishing House and Springer Publishing Company for their recognition of the book, which makes our experience and knowledge more accessible and helpful to other patients and people engaged in pursuit of preventing and treating COVID-19.

Wuhan, China
April 19, 2020

Fanjun Cheng
Yu Zhang

Contents

List of Contributors

Xuefeng Cai, M Med Department of Pharmacy, Union Hospital, Tongji Medical College of Huazhong University of Science and Technology, Wuhan, China

Hui Chen, PhD, MD Department of Obstetrics and Gynaecology, Union Hospital, Tongji Medical College, Huazhong University of Science and Technology, Wuhan, China

Rui Chen, PhD, MD Department of Integrated Traditional Chinese Medicine and Western Medicine, Union Hospital, Tongji Medical College, Huazhong University of Science and Technology, Wuhan, China

Fanjun Cheng Department of Internal Medicine, Union Hospital, Tongji Medical College of Huazhong University of Science and Technology, Wuhan, China

Yunzhou Fan, PhD, MD Department of Nosocomial Infection Management, Union Hospital, Tongji Medical College, Huazhong University of Science and Technology, Wuhan, China

Zhaohui Fu, PhD, MD Critical Care Medicine, Union Hospital, Tongji Medical College, Huazhong University of Science and Technology, Wuhan, China

Yong Gao, PhD, MD Department of Orthopaedics, Union Hospital, Tongji Medical College, Huazhong University of Science and Technology, Wuhan, China

Xiaodan Han, MSc Department of Medical Office, Union Hospital, Tongji Medical College, Huazhong University of Science and Technology, Wuhan, China

Yu Hu, PhD, MD Institute of Hematology, Union Hospital, Tongji Medical College, Huazhong University of Science and Technology, Wuhan, China

Li Jiang Department of Nosocomial Infection Management, Union Hospital, Tongji Medical College, Huazhong University of Science and Technology, Wuhan, China

Yan Jin, M Med Emergency Department, Union Hospital, Tongji Medical College, Huazhong University of Science and Technology, Wuhan, China

Yuncheng Li, PhD, MD Department of Otorhinolaryngology, Union Hospital, Tongji Medical College, Huazhong University of Science and Technology, Wuhan, China

Qian Liu, M Med Department of Nosocomial Infection Management, Union Hospital, Tongji Medical College, Huazhong University of Science and Technology, Wuhan, China

Shi Liu, PhD, MD Division of Gastroenterology, Union Hospital, Tongji Medical College, Huazhong University of Science and Technology, Wuhan, China

Yong Liu, PhD, MD Department of Orthopaedics, Union Hospital, Tongji Medical College, Huazhong University of Science and Technology, Wuhan, China

Jian Luo, M Med Department of Nursing, Union Hospital, Tongji Medical College, Huazhong University of Science and Technology, Wuhan, China

Ying Su, PhD, MD Department of Neurology, Union Hospital, Tongji Medical College, Huazhong University of Science and Technology, Wuhan, China

Yuyong Su, M Med Department of Pharmacy, Union Hospital, Tongji Medical College of Huazhong University of Science and Technology, Wuhan, China

Peng Sun, PhD, MD Department of Emergency Medicine, Union Hospital, Tongji Medical College, Huazhong University of Science and Technology, Wuhan, China

Hongbo Wang, PhD, MD Department of Obstetrics and Gynaecology, Union Hospital, Tongji Medical College, Huazhong University of Science and Technology, Wuhan, China

Hua Wang Hospital Logistics Management, Union Hospital, Tongji Medical College, Huazhong University of Science and Technology, Wuhan, China

Jing Wang, PhD, MD Department of Ultrasound, Union Hospital, Tongji Medical College, Huazhong University of Science and Technology, Wuhan, China

Yadan Wang, PhD, MD Institute of Hematology, Union Hospital, Tongji Medical College, Huazhong University of Science and Technology, Wuhan, China

Weimin Xiao, MD Department of Anesthesiology, Union Hospital, Tongji Medical College, Huazhong University of Science and Technology, Wuhan, China

Mingxing Xie, PhD, MD Department of Ultrasound, Union Hospital, Tongji Medical College, Huazhong University of Science and Technology, Wuhan, China

Hui Xing, M Med Department of Clinical Laboratory, Union Hospital, Tongji Medical College, Huazhong University of Science and Technology, Wuhan, China

Lian Yang, PhD, MD Department of Radiology, Union Hospital, Tongji Medical College, Huazhong University of Science and Technology, Wuhan, China

Jianchu Zhang, PhD, MD Department of Respiratory and Critical Care Medicine, Union Hospital, Tongji Medical College, Huazhong University of Science and Technology, Wuhan, China

Xiaomeng Zhang, PhD, MD Department of Otolaryngology, Union Hospital, Tongji Medical College, Huazhong University of Science and Technology, Wuhan, China

Yong Zhang, PhD, MD Department of Hepatobiliary Surgery, Union Hospital, Tongji Medical College, Huazhong University of Science and Technology, Wuhan, China

Yu Zhang Department of Pharmacy, Union Hospital, Tongji Medical College of Huazhong University of Science and Technology, Wuhan, China

Fang Zheng, PhD, MD Department of Pediatrics, Union Hospital, Tongji Medical College, Huazhong University of Science and Technology, Wuhan, China

Qingtang Zhu, PhD, MD Department of Microsurgery, Orthopaedic Trauma and Hand Surgery, The First Affiliated Hospital, Sun Yat-sen University, Guangzhou, China

English Editing Team

Anbang Cheng Institute of Environmental Engineering, The University of Melbourne, Melbourne, Australia

Zhongbo Hu, PhD, MD Rainbow Babies and Children's Hospital Case Western Reserve University, Cleveland, OH, USA

Mu Hu, Solon, OH, USA

Ziwei Zhang, MA Department of Comprehensive Management, Union Hospital, Tongji Medical College, Huazhong University of Science and Technology, Wuhan, China

Emergency System of Designated Hospital for COVID-19

1

Yong Gao, Yuncheng Li, Jian Luo, Hua Wang, Ying Su, Hui Chen, Xiaodan Han, and Hongbo Wang

Contents

The corresponding author of Sect. 1.1 is Yong Gao, Email: docgao@163.com
The corresponding author of Sect. 1.2 is Yungcheng Li, Email: 912485466@qq.com
The corresponding author of Sect. 1.3 is Ying Su, Email: suying0110@126.com
The corresponding author of Sect. 1.4 is Hui Chen, Email: chinachen67@hust.edu.cn
The corresponding author of Sect. 1.5 is Yungcheng Li, Email: 912485466@qq.com

---

Y. Gao (✉)
Department of Orthopaedics, Union Hospital, Tongji Medical College, Huazhong University of Science and Technology, Wuhan, China

Y. Li
Department of Otorhinolaryngology, Union Hospital, Tongji Medical College, Huazhong University of Science and Technology, Wuhan, China

J. Luo
Department of Nursing, Union Hospital, Tongji Medical College, Huazhong University of Science and Technology, Wuhan, China

H. Wang
Hospital Logistics Management, Union Hospital, Tongji Medical College, Huazhong University of Science and Technology, Wuhan, China

Y. Su
Department of Neurology, Union Hospital, Tongji Medical College, Huazhong University of Science and Technology, Wuhan, China

H. Chen · H. Wang
Department of Obstetrics and Gynaecology, Union Hospital, Tongji Medical College, Huazhong University of Science and Technology, Wuhan, China
e-mail: chinachen67@hust.edu.cn

X. Han
Department of Medical Office, Union Hospital, Tongji Medical College, Huazhong University of Science and Technology, Wuhan, China

F. Cheng, Y. Zhang (eds.), *The Clinical Diagnosis and Treatment for New Coronavirus Pneumonia*, https://doi.org/10.1007/978-981-15-5975-4_1

1.1 Emergency Organizations and Their Responsibilities

Yong Gao

1.1.1 Establishment of Emergency Medical Department

Yong Gao

Under the guidance of the National Health Commission of the People's Republic of China, the Emergency Medical Department is established and formed by the medical administration experts from the national medical teams with the objective of "making every effort to improve the recovery rate and reduce the mortality rate" and upholding the working principle of "joint consultation, united consensus, concerted effort and rapid implementation." It is convened by the medical administration departments of designated hospitals in order to carry out the work focusing on the implementation of core medical system and the improvement of treatment, and its core responsibilities are as follows:

1. Plan, organize, coordinate, and control the whole process of medical activities in the hospital, maintain a high-quality and efficient operation of the medical system, and make the medical activities at the best state by focusing on the management objectives.
2. Concentrate on severe and critical cases; establish a four-level quality control system: medical groups—ward area—district-hospital, and strengthen the supervision and assessment to secure the implementation of the core medical system and provide a systemic guarantee to enhance the diagnosis and treatment quality of severe and critical patients.
3. Thoroughly discuss and analyze within a group about difficult and complicated cases, as well as severe, critical, and death cases; sum up the experience of successful treatment, unite the consensus on diagnosis, treatment and management, and actively promote the application.

4. Coordinate and solve the difficulties and problems found during the practice of clinical and medical technical departments, organize, and participate in the grand rescue and consultation of the whole hospital.
5. Grasp the basic medical information of the hospital accurately, summarize, and submit the medical brief report of the hospital.
6. Establish and improve the report, investigation, and handling mechanism of medical adverse events.
7. Take in charge of the daily management of the fever clinic and the medical treatment of severe urgent patients in the hospital.
8. Complete other jobs assigned by the epidemic prevention headquarters.

1.1.2 Innovation of Emergency Medical Administration

Yuncheng Li

1.1.2.1 Establishment of the Discussion System for Emergency Response to Difficult and Complicated cases, as well as Severe, Critical, and Death Cases

The establishment of the discussion system for difficult and complicated, severe, critical, and death cases shall be based on the actual situation and implemented by different levels in multiple ways during epidemic prevention and control. The participants shall include frontline medical staff at all levels, members of expert groups in each ward area, directors of ward areas, district principals, members of the hospital expert group, and personnel of the Emergency Medical Department. For the COVID-19 patients to be analyzed with other serious systemic diseases and cannot be provided with professional and technical services in the ward area/district, suggestions can be made to the Emergency Medical Department 2 h in advance, and the Emergency Medical Department shall coordinate and allocate relevant experts. The number of participants in the discussion shall be properly limited based on the principle of being highly capable, efficient, and problem-solving. Encourage all medical teams to tackle the problems with rear professional and technical forces of their respective hospitals.

Set up a three-level discussion system of ward area—district—hospital for cases. The case discussion at the ward level shall be led by the ward area director, and the discussion time and frequency shall not be limited, but shall meet the requirements of the core medical system and be timely reported to the Emergency Medical Department; for the cases requiring discussion at the district level, the ward area director shall prepare the reporting and discussion materials, and the district principal shall determine the frequency and participants; for the cases requiring discussion at the hospital level, the leader of the expert group shall organize the discussion by at least once a week.

The ward area director shall deliver the case materials submitted for discussion at the district and hospital levels to the participants in advance and keep a medical record. The Emergency Medical Department shall dispatch personnel to participate in the discussion and keep a work record.

The subjects of case discussion include death cases, critical and severe cases, difficult and complicated cases as well as some cases participating in specific non-double-blind clinical studies. It is also suggested to include the critical and severe cases with successful treatment to provide learning experiences and submit the refined views and methods to the Treatment Expert Group of National Health Commission for real-time sharing.

1.1.2.2 Continuous Optimization of the Quality Control Mechanism of Emergency Medical Services

Establish an expert group for the diagnosis and treatment of difficult and complicated, severe and critical COVID-19 cases to conduct a unified assessment and checklist management of all COVID-19 patients admitted to the hospital, and individualize the treatment plan on the basis of national guidelines to improve the success rate of rescue.

Periodically study and evaluate the medical quality status of each ward area and put forward suggestions for improvement to the hospital executives.

Establish a joint expert group and a discussion system for severe and critical patients. Carry out multidisciplinary treatment (MDT) for rarely seen difficult and complicated cases, invite members of the national expert group to give guidance, and adjust the existing treatment plan through case discussion and MDT to form a comprehensive treatment plan.

Develop a reporting system for the expected death of severe and critical patients, with the purpose of strengthening the management of severe and critical patients. Provide early warning for the potential deadly cases and make active and reasonable intervention, strengthen the responsibilities and timely revise the treatment plan.

1.1.3 Emergency Nursing Management

Jian Luo

1.1.3.1 Establishment of Emergency Nursing Management System

1.1.3.1.1 Set Up an Emergency Nursing Command System

Quickly establish an emergency management system mainly including the nursing department of the hospital and head nurse of the ward area. The director of the nursing department is fully responsible for the work deployment and implementation, designating the nursing staff of the hospital to be responsible for the clinical nursing quality, nursing safety, and allocation of nursing human resources; the head nurse of each ward area shall ensure the execution of all measures.

The director of the nursing department shall timely discover, guide the processing and report various emergencies in case of a sudden outbreak, effectively coordinate with medical treatment, inspection, and logistics departments to solve specific problems in clinical nursing and ensure the treatment of patients.

The director of the nursing department shall strengthen communication with the nursing directors of the national medical teams, establish the emergency nursing department and hold regular meetings; the head nurse of the ward area shall closely cooperate with the national medical teams to mutually complete the nursing services of the ward area.

1.1.3.2 Reasonable Allocation of Nursing Human Resources

1.1.3.2.1 Assess the Human Resource Allocation

Sort out the epidemic prevention, control posts, and establish a highly capable and efficient human resource echelon for emergency nursing. Quickly allocate nurses to their posts according to their age, level, professional title, specialized technical level, and in combination with post needs, so as to maximize their talents and efficiency [1].

1.1.3.2.2 Arrange Working Hours Appropriately

Looking at the fact that COVID-19 is an infectious disease mainly transmitted through the respiratory tract [2] and the nursing staff works with great physical exertion under the strict protective equipment, the length of each shift shall be controlled between 4 and 6 h to ensure safety.

1.1.3.2.3 Active Reserve of Nursing Staff

Companion is not allowed in the isolation ward. The treatment:living care of patients as well as partial infection work of the hospital are all undertaken by the nurses. Sufficient nursing human resources shall be provided with perhaps 3 times the standard for nurses in general wards.

1.1.3.2.4 Integration of Human Resources and Scheduling Dynamically and Flexibly

The nursing department shall actively communicate with each national medical team and reasonably allocate human resources according to the number of nursing staff in each national medical team to ensure the relative balance of human resources in each ward area [3]. When scheduling the nursing staff, it is advised to reserve a spare shift throughout the day to replace the nursing staffs who are urgently withdrawn from the isolation ward area due to physical discomfort.

1.1.3.3 Formulate Relevant Systems, Processes, and Emergency Plans to Ensure the Safety and Efficiency of Nursing Work

Develop the nursing process, preexamination and triage process, vital signs checking and nursing process, specimen collection and management process, disease observation and nursing process, nutrition support and nursing process, patient outcome and nursing process, the process of medical staff accompanying the patient to go out for examination, patient admission and referral workflow, ward disinfection workflow, rescue and nursing workflow for critical and severe patients, and psychological assessment and counseling process for COVID-19 patients, etc.

Relevant nursing systems and processes: Post the responsibilities of nursing staff in each isolation ward area, the work responsibilities of each shift, the management systems and requirements on staff, the entry and exit process of isolation cabin, the physical condition monitoring process of nursing staff and the standard for emergency exit from isolation cabin, etc. Ensure that the nursing staffs are supported in their work.

1.1.3.3.1 Emergency Plan

Patient-related emergency plans: Emergency plans to prevent falling from bed, for patients leaving without permission, for patients with suicidal ideation, and for accidents in the use of infusion pump, ventilator, monitor and defibrillator, etc.

Nursing-related emergency plans: Emergency plans for physical discomfort, needle injury, damaged personal protective equipment, excessive moisture, and fall prevention in the isolation cabin.

1.1.3.4 Preparation of Ward Environment, Instruments, Equipment, and Materials

1.1.3.4.1 Strict Partition and Reasonable Arrangement of Wards

The isolation ward area is strictly divided into the contaminated area, the semi-contaminated area, and the clean area. There is no overlap in the three areas, with unified and eye-catching signs in each area.

Clean area: Refers to the area kept away from patients and pathogenic bacteria. There are changing rooms, duty rooms, warehouses, restrooms, bathrooms, and dispensing rooms for medical staff in the clean area.

Semi-contaminated area: Refers to the area that may be contaminated by pathogenic microorganisms, such as internal corridors, doctor's and nurse's offices, and treatment rooms.

Contaminated area: Refers to the area often in contact with patients and contaminated by pathogenic microorganisms, including wards, bathrooms, and toilets for patients. Each isolation ward area is equipped with 30–50 beds, single rooms for suspected patients, double or triple rooms for confirmed patients, and bedside treatment facilities such as oxygen and suction equipment as well as calling and intercom equipment in the ward. All wards are equipped with independent toilets, defecators, showers, hand washing facilities, etc.

Separate the clean and contaminated routes with no overlap in strict accordance with the flow of people and materials.

Arrange the work areas of medical staff according to the workflow: clean area → semi-contaminated area → contaminated area and set a pass-through changing station at the entrance of the work area at each level.

1.1.3.4.2 Material Preparation

The emergency nursing department shall actively make overall planning and apply for the use of various essential materials.

Basic materials: Bed sheets, quilt covers, medical waste bags, cleaning carts, rags, mops, disinfectants, measuring cups, buckets, air disinfectors, etc.

Protective materials: Surgical gowns, gloves, KN95/N95 masks, surgical masks, protective suits, isolation gowns or waterproof aprons, special shoe covers, goggles, protective masks, caps, etc. [4].

Rescue materials: Powered air-purifying respirators, ventilators, ECG monitors, defibrillators, micro-infusion pumps, injection pumps, emergency ambulances, CRRT, etc.

Special materials: Special materials for ward areas shall be registered and claimed by specially assigned persons in clean areas to ensure rational use and avoid unnecessary waste.

1.1.3.5 Training and Assessment for Strengthening Prejob Knowledge and Skills

1.1.3.5.1 Training Content

The training shall be jointly completed by the emergency nursing department and the ward area, including the epidemiological characteristics of COVID-19, prevention and control systems and measures, operation specifications for nursing, emergency plans for occupational exposure, collection and transport of specimens, disinfection and isolation knowledge, correct procedures for putting on and taking off protective equipment, workflow of each shift, application of common rescue operating skills and equipment, nervousness adjustment before entering the cabin, and physical adaptability training.

1.1.3.5.2 Training Method

Combine the multi-session centralized training (the trainees shall wear masks, with a seat spacing >1 m) with network training (WeChat platform and 317hu learning platform) to achieve comprehensive, all-inclusive, hierarchical, and content-rich training management [5].

1.1.3.5.3 Strict Assessment

Uniformly assess the trainees and record the results after the training to discover the problems in a timely manner sum up experience and improve the practical coping skills.

1.1.3.6 Implementation of Nursing Quality Management

Set up a nursing quality control squad to go to each ward area every day for strict supervision, timely report problems and urge the department to complete rectification as soon as possible, to ensure the quality and safety of nursing.

Implement the prevention and control measures for infection in the ward, inform hospitalized patients to wear surgical masks in a unified and correct manner, and carry out personal hygiene; assist the infection control department of the hospital to supervise the quality of medical waste treatment, cleaning, and disinfection of cleaning personnel; the head nurse in each ward area shall carry out basic supervision and management through on-site inspection and questions, etc. to ensure the implementation of prevention and control work for infection in the hospital.

In order to continuously improve the nursing level of critical and severe patients, information exchange meetings are held regularly every Friday afternoon to share the management, treatment, and nursing experience of critical and severe patients with national medical teams to achieve mutual promotion.

As respiratory support is the major management for COVID-19 patients, it is of great importance to standardize the nursing of oxygen therapy in designated hospitals. The respiratory rate, oxygen saturation, and arterial blood gas analysis result of the patient shall be closely monitored, and appropriate mode of oxygen administration and oxygen flow shall be selected according to the degree of hypoxia in the patient.

Skin care and management: Skin assessment is included in the first nursing assessment for patients admitted within 2 h, and preventive measures shall be taken for patients with high risks by Braden score; for patients screened with stage III or above pressure ulcers before admission to the hospital, the wound team shall be timely organized for wound assessment and dressing change.

1.1.3.7 Strengthening of Psychological Nursing and Humanistic Care for Patients

Severe/Critical COVID-19 patients admitted to the hospital shall receive management and treatment in isolation according to the laws. Patients' anxiety about the prognosis of the disease, their fear of death, and their self-blame for the infection of their involved family members will result in psychological reactions of stress, anxiety, and panic to different degrees. Therefore, the nursing staff shall use the *Psychological Rating Scale for COVID-19 Patients* to conduct a preliminary screening of hospitalized patients and perform targeted psychological counseling according to the results. Helping patients to maintain a positive attitude is vital in disease treatment and rehabilitation.

For the patients with serious psychological problems and poor counseling effect, the ward area shall report to the emergency nursing department that shall select appropriate personnel to provide psychological counseling for the patients with applicable methods, to relieve them from negative emotions, and make them actively cooperate with the treatment and nursing care.

Humanistic care and multiple measures: The nurses in the ward area can take the initiative to act as the "temporary family members" of patients to make them feel the care of loved ones. "Temporary family members" refer to that a nurse claims a patient, understands the need of the patient, solves the difficulties in the patient's life, helps the patient communicate with the doctor for treatment, and assumes the responsibility of accompanying and enlightening the patient; a wishing wall can also be set up in the ward area to let nurses and patients write down their wishes for mutual encouragement and blessing.

1.1.3.8 Pay Attention to the Physical and Mental Health of Nursing Staff in the Isolation Ward Area

Provide a channel for nursing staff to relieve their psychological pressure. Timely understand the psychological status of nursing staff in the ward area and provide psychological counseling for nurses with psychological difficulties. Specific measures include but are not limited to warming, understanding, and encouraging messages from head nurses, looking for suitable opportunities for off-duty nurses to vent their negative emotions/get encouragement and support to restore their fighting capacity, carrying out psychological training to distribute their energy, physical strength, and attention rationally and carrying out psychological intervention on nursing staff with great psychological pressure [6].

Establish a guarantee and incentive system for anti-epidemic nursing staff. Provide good food, accommodation, and transportation for nursing staff in isolation ward areas, provide anti-epidemic subsidies, living materials support, rest plan and other measures [7], give praise, and policy inclination to nursing staff involved in the treatment of COVID-19, and publicize advanced nursing deeds/write nurse anti-epidemic stories in an appropriate way to spread positive energy.

1.1.4 Emergency Logistics Management in Designated Hospitals

Hua Wang

After being designated as the designated hospital of COVID-19, the logistics management of medical institutions will face a new working situation. The logistics work must ensure that the patient treatment can be smoothly carried out and a strengthened logistics operation management system will be formed as soon as possible.

1.1.4.1 Promote the Leading Decision-making Position of Logistics Support Organizations

In designated hospitals, the dean of administrative logistics shall be designated to be responsible for logistics support, and a logistics support department composed of existing logistics personnel, social workers, and volunteers shall be set up to carry out the work.

The logistics department can set up the following teams according to the situation to ensure all logistics tasks during the epidemic prevention and control of COVID-19.

1.1.4.1.1 Logistics Outreach Team

Responsible for contacting the leaders of the hospital in charge and receiving the government anti-epidemic materials and social donation materials and other related affairs.

1.1.4.1.2 Hydroelectric Kinetic Energy Gas Team

Responsible for the water and electricity kinetic energy protection and the gas support required for patient treatment during the epidemic period.

1.1.4.1.3 Catering Team

Responsible for the food processing and distribution of all staff and patients during the epidemic period, with each aspect of the work meeting the requirements of biosecurity hospital infection protection.

1.1.4.1.4 Disinfection and Cleaning Team

Perform effective sanitation practices and waste removal in various areas in accordance with the requirements of Class A infectious diseases.

1.1.4.1.5 Facilities and Equipment Team

Ensure the fitting of the requirements of medical rescue equipment and life-supporting equipment.

1.1.4.1.6 Security and Fire Safety Team

Responsible for the management of all passages in the designated hospital area and the safety management of patients and assisting in completing the fire safety work.

1.2 Basic Medical Quality Management

Yuncheng Li and Xiaodan Han

1.2.1 Ward Rounding System

Ward rounding system [8] is a routine work for medical staff at all levels to understand and grasp the changes of patients' conditions at any time through the inspection of hospitalized COVID-19 patients, and is the key to ensure timely and effective treatment for COVID-19 patients. In addition to resident doctor rounds, countries and regions can implement ward rounding system according to the regulations of local health administrative departments, which can only be strengthened but not weakened.

1.2.1.1 Three-level Physician Ward Rounding System

The deputy chief physician or above of the ward area shall be responsible. The deputy chief physician shall make ward rounds at least twice a week and may increase the number of rounds according to the needs of patients. In case of critical and difficult patients, he/she shall be on call.

1.2.1.2 Attending Physician Ward Rounding System

The professional and technical personnel of attending physicians and above make ward rounds at least once a day.

1.2.2 On Duty System

Medical institutions shall establish a hospital-wide medical duty system, including clinical, medical and nursing departments, and logistics departments that provide diagnosis and treatment support, and specify the duties of each duty post and the qualifications and number of duty personnel. All diagnosis and treatment activities during duty must be recorded in the medical record in time [8].

1.2.2.1 First-line Doctor on Duty System

Including resident doctors, attending doctors with low seniority, refresher doctors, and graduate candidates with clinical experience and practicing qualifications of doctors in our hospital; the doctor on duty is responsible for the instant medical work and situation of the patient, timely examining and filling the medical records for patients admitted to hospital urgently, and giving necessary medical treatment.

1.2.2.2 Second-line Doctor Duty System

Including senior doctors with attending physician or above in the hospital; the second-line doctor on duty must stick to his/her post in the department and must not leave his/her post; the second-line doctor on duty must keep the duty phone unblocked, and shall tell the on-duty doctor and nurse in the ward area where to go when leaving the ward area due to necessary work.

1.2.3 Consultation System

Due to the need of comprehensive diagnosis and management, the activity paradigm for medical staff outside the ward area or outside the institution to assist in finalizing the diagnosis and treatment opinions or providing diagnosis and treatment services is called consultation system [8].

1.2.3.1 General Consultation

During the process of diagnosis and treatment in each ward area in the hospital, ordinary consultation can be applied for when relevant departments are required to assist in diagnosis and treatment according to the patient's condition or relevant regulations. Invited departments/ward areas shall give consultation opinions or suggestions within 24 h.

1.2.3.2 Emergency Consultation

In the treatment or rescue of acute and critical patients, emergency consultation can be applied for urgent and difficult problems that must be solved by consultation. The second-line doctors on duty of the invited department/ward area must arrive at the consultation ward area within 10 min. Under special circumstances, consultation services can be completed by telephone or network.

1.2.3.3 Surgical Consultation

In case of serious situations or difficulty in operation, surgical consultation can be applied for when higher-level doctors or relevant experts need to participate in the operation and rescue.

1.2.3.4 Ordinary Consultation Mode

Consultation in the ward area: Proposed by the attending physician and attended by relevant personnel in the ward area convened by the ward area director.

Consultation in the district: Proposed by the ward area director and participated by other departments in the hospital.

Consultation in the hospital: Proposed by the district director and participated by multiple districts and professionals.

Consultation outside the hospital: Proposed by the ward area director and participated by other hospitals outside the hospital by invitation of the medical department.

Teleconsultation: proposed by the ward area director and participated by other ward areas/hospitals outside the ward area/hospital through the teleconsultation system by invitation of the medical department.

1.3 Admission and Treatment Process of COVID-19

Ying Su

1.3.1 Principles for Admission and Treatment of COVID-19 Patients [9]

Simplify admission procedures, reduce the flow of patients in the hospital, register patient information with legal name, and achieve admission without card (medical insurance card).

Patients will be allocated uniformly by the allocation team of medical department according to the patient's condition and the beds availability in the ward area. Patients are not allowed to be admitted to each ward area by the ward themselves.

In general, all patients are admitted and treated in a single room. If beds are insufficient, 2–3 confirmed cases can be received and treated in one unit, and the suspected cases should be admitted and treated in a single room.

It is suggested that mild and severe patients should be admitted and treated separately and critically ill patients should be allocated in ICU uniformly.

NCP patients with similar underlying diseases are admitted and treated in the same ward area, which is convenient for special diagnosis and management of underlying diseases.

1.3.2 Process for Admission and Treatment of COVID-19 Patients

The allocation team of medical department (hereinafter referred to as the allocation team) collects the information of the admitted patients (name, sex, age, contact information, ID number, home address, and medical insurance information), evaluates the patient's health condition, and determines the admission ward area and beds.

The allocation team informs the nurse station in the ward area to prepare for receiving and treatment and basic information of the patients.

The allocation team informs the assistance center to handle the legal name registration and admission procedures.

The allocation team informs 120 ambulances to send the patients directly to the designated ward area of the inpatient department.

1.4 Medical Treatment Process for Pregnant Women

Hui Chen and Hongbo Wang

Hospitals shall set up fever clinic and clinic assistance center to facilitate the hospitalization and management for febrile pregnant and lying-in women. Pregnant women with fever, cough, chest distress, runny nose, diarrhea, and other symptoms shall first go to fever clinic for treatment under the guidance of special personnel.

Outpatient workup shall include the following items: Chest CT, complete blood count, novel coronavirus nasopharyngeal swab or blood virus nucleic acid assay, novel coronavirus blood antibody assay (IgM and IgG), 3-item respiratory tract virus assay, and screening for A/H1N1 influenza.

For pregnant women with confirmed or suspected COVID-19, the staff of the clinic assistance center shall contact the ward for admission and management. For hospitals without an assistance center, the outpatient managing physician shall directly contact the ward for admission and management. The pregnant and lying-in cases with suspected or confirmed diagnosis of COVID-19 shall be reported according to the regulations of epidemic of infectious diseases.

Hospitals with isolated obstetrics department are designated hospitals for receiving and treating pregnant women with COVID-19. They do not undertake prenatal examination and postpartum health care for pregnant and lying-in women without COVID-19.

If febrile pregnant women have vaginal bleeding, paroxysmal abdominal pain, and other obstetric labor or abortion clinical manifestations, treat separately according to the following two situations:

1. Fever clinics and isolated obstetrics departments shall inform patients of the risk of cross-infection during hospitalization without being confirmed as COVID-19, which may endanger the safety of pregnant women and fetuses. If patients

clearly indicate that they know and bear all the effects of the viral infection on their health, they can be admitted to isolated obstetrics department for observation and treatment.

2. Patients with confirmed or suspected of COVID-19 shall be admitted to the isolated obstetrics department for management.

For pregnant cases with positive nucleic acid testing, there are indications for admission and management in isolated obstetrics department regardless of gestational age and birth sign.

For pregnant cases who have no indications for emergency obstetric care, no pneumonia manifestations and no novel coronavirus testing, the designated hospitals will not accept them. Clinic service shall guide them to other hospitals for obstetric care.

1.5 Disposal Process of Remains of Patients with COVID-19

Yuncheng Li

According to the regulations of *Disposal Process of Remains of Patients with COVID-19 (Trial) from* the Wuhan COVID-19 Prevention and Control Headquarters Office, the remains of suspected and confirmed patients with COVID-19 shall be disposed according to the following process [10]:

1. Within 30 min after the death of the patient with COVID-19, the medical staff shall:
   (a) Notify family members to come to the hospital and go through the formalities.
   (b) Issue the medical death certificate to family members by physician, in which the funeral cremation couplet is handed over from the ward area to the funeral parlor staff.
   (c) Complete the disposal of hygiene and epidemic prevention of remains: Medical staffs use cotton balls containing disinfectants to block the cavity. After disinfection, a 1-layer sealed body bag is used for the first sealing. After repeated disinfection, a 1-layer sealed body bag is used for the second sealing. It is forbidden to open the remains after sealing.
   (d) Confirm with the family members as soon as possible in the *Receiving Registration Form of Remains* and obtain signature.
   (e) After the remains are transferred, complete the disinfection of the surroundings according to the hospital's infection requirements.
2. If the patient's relatives are unable to be present, in addition to the above actions, medical staff shall:
   (a) Directly contact the police station in the jurisdiction area to provide the identity information of the deceased, the retained family information, and contact information for inquiry and review by the police station.

(b) If the patient has valuables, such as wallets, bank cards, and other belongings; seal them after disinfection, mark with patient information, and then store them.
(c) If the police confirm that the patient's family members cannot be contacted, or if the family members refuse to transfer the remains, inform the hospital security department to coordinate with public security office for disposal.
(d) The remains shall not be stored, visited, or held funeral activities such as farewell ceremonies. It is strictly prohibited to open the sealed body bag during the whole process.

References

1. Wang L, Xiaochun P, Le K, et al. Functions and deployment of nursing department in response to COVID-19 epidemic. Chinese Nursing Research. 2020;34(4):571–2.
2. Al-Tawfiq JA, Auwaerter PG. Health care associated infections: the hallmark of Middle East respiratory syndrome coronavirus with review of the literature. J Hosp Infect. 2019;101(1):20–9.
3. Mei F, Wu Y, Wu X, et al. Construction of Nursing Team of First-line Support Medical Team against COVID-19. Chin J Respir Crit Care Med. 2020;19(2):1–4.
4. National Health Committee of the PRC. Guidelines on the scope of use of common medical protective equipment in infection prevention and control against COVID-19 [EB/OL]. (2020-01-27) [2020-01-28].
5. Qiong Y, Zhang L, Wu L, et al. Emergency training and effect of anti-epidemic nurses against COVID-19. J Nurs (China). 2020;27(6):52–5.
6. Chen M, Fang H, Li L. Emergency management strategy of nursing human resources in designated hospitals for COVID-19 patients. Mod Clin Nurs. 2020;19(2):1–4.
7. Chen J, Shi J, Zhao X. Thoughts on effective psychological assistance during the epidemic period of COVID-19. J Tongji Univ. 2020;41(1):5–8.
8. National Health Commission of the PRC. Key points of core system for medical quality and safety. April 18, 2018. http://www.ncis.cn/page.jsp?id=191&mod=100
9. Interim measures for prevention and control of COVID-19 in Wuhan city. http://wjw.wuhan.gov.cn/front/web/showDetail/2020020209339
10. Medical Treatment Group of Wuhan COVID-19 Prevention and Control Headquarters. Notice on further strengthening the transfer and disposal of remains of patients infected with COVID-19 (including suspected cases), February 2, 2020.

Hospital Infection Prevention and Control Against COVID-19

2

Li Jiang, Qian Liu, Yunzhou Fan, Yan Jin, Fanjun Cheng, and Yong Gao

Contents

The corresponding author of Sect. 2.1 is Qian Liu, Email: 370853348@qq.com
The corresponding author of Sect. 2.2 is Qian Liu, Email: 370853348@qq.com
The corresponding author of Sect. 2.3 is Yunzhou Fan, Email: fyz88033@126.com
The corresponding author of Sect. 2.4 is Yunzhou Fan, Email: fyz88033@126.com
The corresponding author of Sect. 2.5 is Yan Jin, Email: yanjin@126.com
The corresponding author of Sect. 2.6 is Yong Gao, Email: docgao@163.com

L. Jiang (✉) · Q. Liu · Y. Fan
Department of Nosocomial Infection Management, Union Hospital, Tongji Medical College, Huazhong University of Science and Technology, Wuhan, China

Y. Jin
Emergency Department, Union Hospital, Tongji Medical College, Huazhong University of Science and Technology, Wuhan, China

F. Cheng
Department of Internal Medicine, Union Hospital, Tongji Medical College of Huazhong University of Science and Technology, Wuhan, China

Y. Gao
Department of Orthopaedics, Union Hospital, Tongji Medical College, Huazhong University of Science and Technology, Wuhan, China

F. Cheng, Y. Zhang (eds.), *The Clinical Diagnosis and Treatment for New Coronavirus Pneumonia*, https://doi.org/10.1007/978-981-15-5975-4_2

2.1 Regional Isolation and Management

Li Jiang, Qian Liu and Yunzhou Fan

2.1.1 Daily Cleaning and Disinfection Process for Public Areas

Cleaning personnel shall wear personal protective equipment according to the regional risk level (referring to the Attachment for the division of risk areas and personal protection requirements).

Cleaning tools shall be prepared, including cleaning trolleys, rags, mops, disinfectants, measuring cups, barrels, and tidying boxes.

Disinfectant shall be prepared: Jianzhisu effervescent tablets can be prepared into 1000 mg/L available chlorine disinfectant. After preparation, disinfectant concentration test paper shall be used to monitor and record the effective concentration. Only after monitoring is qualified can the disinfectant be used. Note: Chlorine-containing disinfectants shall be ready for use, and the use time shall not exceed 24 h.

Cleaning and disinfection of areas with special infected patients and terminal disinfection shall be carried out under the guidance of professionals.

Cleaning and Disinfection of Public Areas

All public areas shall be cleaned and regularly disinfected three times a day, especially in frequent contact areas, such as all inner surfaces of elevators, seats, and registration and payment machines.

During wiping, the surface of objects shall be cleaned and disinfected in the order from clean to dirty. Wipe the relatively less contacted environmental surface first, then the frequently contacted environmental surface, and finally the floor inside the toilet and the surface of objects used. Replace a rag after wiping the surface of one object.

The ground is wiped with chlorine-containing disinfectant for the duration of 30 min.

When the surface of the object or ground is contaminated by the blood and body fluid of the patient, cleaning personnel shall wear gloves. First remove visible contamination, contaminants with moisture absorption methods (high-quality paper towel is recommended), then wipe with chlorine-containing disinfectant, and finally with clean water after 30 min.

The special elevator for specimen transportation and COVID-19 patient transfer shall be disinfected frequently, at least three times a day. Chlorine-containing disinfectant can be used to wipe the bottom and surface of the cart for 30 min, and then the air supply system can be turned on for 1 h before use of the special elevator.

Handling of Cleaning Tools After Use

Rags and mops: soak in chlorine-containing disinfectant for 30 min; clean and dry for standby.

Cleaning trolley: push it back to the disposal room after use, wipe the trolley with chlorine-containing disinfectant, and then wipe with clean water to remove the residual disinfectant for later use.

Contamination Risk Grade in Public Areas

Low-risk areas: areas where there are basically no patients, such as administrative departments, conference rooms, and medical record rooms.

Moderate-risk areas: functional examination rooms and other areas.

High-risk areas: fever clinic and isolation ward.

2.1.2 Cleaning and Disinfection System for Fever Clinic

Disposable diagnosis and treatment equipment shall be selected as far as possible, non-disposable diagnosis and treatment equipment shall be first sterilized by pressure steam, and non-heat resistant articles can be sterilized by chemical disinfectant or low-temperature sterilization equipment.

It is suggested to choose effective disinfectants such as iodophor, chlorine-containing disinfectant, and hydrogen peroxide disinfectant for hand and skin or ABHR for wiping and disinfection.

The surface of objects and ground shall be cleaned and disinfected regularly three times a day. Disinfection shall be carried out in time in case of contamination.

Ventilation (including natural ventilation and mechanical ventilation) measures can be taken to maintain indoor air circulation. Ventilation shall be conducted two to three times a day for no less than 30 min each time, or circulating air disinfecting machine shall be used for disinfection.

Ground and wall: when there are visible contaminants, the contaminants shall be completely removed before disinfection. When there is no visible contaminant, 1000 mg/L chlorine-containing disinfectant can be used to wipe or spray for disinfection. Disinfection time shall be not less than 30 min.

Surface of objects: when there are visible contaminants on the surface of diagnosis and treatment facilities and equipment, bed fences, bedside tables, furniture, door handles, and household items, the contaminants shall be completely removed before disinfection. When there are no visible contaminants, chlorine-containing disinfectant shall be used to spray, wipe, or soak for disinfection. Wipe clean with clean water after 30 min.

Treatment of contaminants (blood, secretions, vomitus, and excreta of patients): A small amount of contaminants can be carefully removed by disposable absorbent materials (such as gauze, rag) dipping with 5000–10,000 mg/L chlorine-containing disinfectant (or disinfectant wipes/dry wipes capable of achieving high-level disinfection). A large amount of contaminants shall be completely covered with disinfectant powder or bleaching powder containing water-absorbing components, or completely covered with disposable absorbent materials, and then sufficient chlorine-containing disinfectant of 5000–10,000 mg/L is poured on the absorbent materials for more than 30 min, and then carefully removed. Avoid contact with contaminants during the cleaning process. The cleaned contaminants shall be disposed of as medical wastes. Patients' excreta, secretions, and vomitus shall be collected in special containers and soaked in chlorine-containing disinfectant of 20,000 mg/L for 2 h according to the ratio of feces to drug of 1:2. After contaminants are removed, the surface of the contaminated environmental objects shall be disinfected. Containers containing contaminants can be soaked in disinfectant containing 5000 mg/L of available chlorine for disinfection for 30 min and then cleaned.

2.1.3 Daily Cleaning and Disinfection System in Isolation Ward Area

Daily cleaning and disinfection of the ward area shall be jointly undertaken by the nursing staff and cleaning personnel of the ward area. The nursing team shall have a disinfection squad every day, specially being responsible for guiding the personal protection of cleaning personnel on duty, and assisting the cleaning personnel in jointly completing the cleaning and disinfection work on that day. The head nurse of the ward area shall be responsible for supervising and implementing the work.

Disposable diagnosis and treatment equipment shall be selected as much as possible. Non-disposable diagnosis and treatment articles shall be first sterilized by pressure steam, and non-heat resistant articles can be sterilized by chemical disinfectant or low-temperature sterilization equipment.

Preparation of Disinfectant (Use Measuring Cup)

Jianzhisu effervescent tablets (500 mg/granule): prepared into 1000 mg/L available chlorine disinfectant.

Preparation method: add 2 tablets of 500 mg/granule in 1 L water and 12 tablets in 6 L water.

After disinfectant is prepared, disinfectant concentration test paper shall be used to monitor and record the effective concentration. Only after the monitoring is qualified can the disinfectant be used. Note: Chlorine-containing disinfectants shall be ready for use, and the use time shall not exceed 24 h.

The surface of objects and ground shall be cleaned and disinfected regularly three times a day. Disinfection shall be carried out in time in case of contamination.

Disinfection Method

Indoor air can be disinfected by ventilation, air disinfecting machine, or ultraviolet ray.

During wiping, the surface of objects shall be cleaned and disinfected in the order from clean to dirty ones. Use chlorine-containing disinfectant containing 1000 mg/L of available chlorine to wipe the relatively less contacted environmental surfaces first, then wipe the frequently contacted environmental surfaces, and finally wipe the floor inside the toilet and the surface of objects used. Replace a piece of rag after wiping the surface of one object, or wipe and disinfect with disposable hydrogen peroxide disinfectant wipes.

The ground is wiped with chlorine-containing disinfectant with an effect of 30 min.

When the surface of the object or ground is obviously contaminated by the blood and body fluid of the patient, cleaning personnel shall wear gloves, first remove visible contaminants with moisture absorption method (high-quality paper towel is recommended), then wipe with chlorine-containing disinfectant containing 1000 mg/L of available chlorine, and wipe with clean water after 30 min.

The empty oxygen cylinder used in the ward area shall be wiped and disinfected with chlorine-containing disinfectant or hydrogen peroxide disinfectant wipes and then transported to the designated position. The humidification bottles are recovered and then sent to the disinfection and supply center for centralized disposal.

The specimen storage box in the ward area shall be wiped with chlorine-containing disinfectant on the inner and outer surfaces three times a day.

Medical waste shall comply with the requirements of *Regulations on Medical Waste Management* and *Measures for Medical Waste Management in Medical and Health Institutions*. Double-layer yellow medical waste collection bags shall be standardized for packing. Another layer of yellow medical waste bags shall be placed on the contaminant elevator for recycling by personnel of temporary storage room.

Handling of Cleaning Tools after Use:

- Rags and mops: soak in disinfectant containing 1000 mg/L available chlorine for 30 min, wash, and dry for standby.
- Cleaning trolley: push it back to the disposal room after use, wipe the trolley with chlorine-containing disinfectant, and then wipe with clean water to remove the residual disinfectant for later use.

2.1.4 Terminal Disinfection System in Isolation Ward Area

Disinfection timing: terminal disinfection refers to thorough disinfection after the source of infection leaves the relevant places, such as disinfection of air, object surface, and ground in the ward after the patient is discharged from hospital, transferred to hospital or died. It shall be ensured that pathogens no longer exist in the places after terminal disinfection and various articles therein. Terminal disinfection objects include contaminants (blood waves, secretions, vomit, excretions, etc.) discharged by cases (suspected cases, confirmed cases) and infected persons (mild cases, asymptomatic infected persons) as well as articles and places that may be contaminated. It is not necessary to carry out large-scale disinfection of outdoor environment (including air). No terminal disinfection is required for places without obvious contaminants where cases and infected persons have stayed temporarily.

Disinfection process: disinfection by hydrogen peroxide sterilizer—routine wiping for cleaning and disinfection-ventilation.

Executor: medical staff on duty in the work area is responsible for terminal disinfection in the area, and the specific executor is assigned by the department.

Disinfection Method:

Close doors and windows, disinfect the air with hydrogen peroxide sterilizer, seal the room for no less than 30 min, and open the window for ventilation.

Ground and wall: when there are visible contaminants, the contaminants shall be completely removed before disinfection. When there are no visible contaminants, 1000 mg/L chlorine-containing disinfectant can be used to wipe or spray for disinfection. Disinfection time shall be not less than 30 min.

Surface of objects: when there are visible contaminants on the surface of diagnosis and treatment facilities and equipment, bed fences, bedside tables, furniture, door handles, household items, etc., the contaminants shall be completely removed before disinfection. When there are no visible contaminants, chlorine-containing disinfectant shall be used to spray, wipe, or soak for disinfection. Wipe and clean with clean water after 30 min.

Treatment of contaminants (blood, secretions, vomitus, and excreta of patients): A small amount of contaminants can be carefully removed by disposable absorbent materials (such as gauze and rag) dipping with 5000–10,000 mg/L chlorine-containing disinfectant (or disinfectant wipes/dry wipes capable of achieving high-level disinfection). A large amount of contaminants shall be completely covered with disinfectant powder or bleaching powder containing water-absorbing components, or completely covered with disposable absorbent materials, and then sufficient chlorine-containing disinfectant of 5000–10,000 mg/L is poured on the absorbent materials for more than 30 min, and then carefully removed. Avoid contact with contaminants during the cleaning process. The cleaned contaminants shall be disposed of as medical wastes. Patients' excreta, secretions, and vomitus shall be collected in special containers and soaked in chlorine-containing disinfectant of 20,000 mg/L for 2 h according to the ratio of feces to drug of 1:2. After contaminants are removed, the surface of the contaminated environmental objects shall be disinfected. Containers containing contaminants can be soaked in disinfectant containing 5000 mg/L of available chlorine for disinfection for 30 min and then cleaned.

Treatment of fabrics: the sheets, quilt covers, and other fabrics used by the patient shall be packaged and sealed with orange soluble packaging bags, marked, and put to the west contaminant ladder, which shall be disinfected and cleaned uniformly by the quilt and clothing warehouse, and handover records shall be made.

Medical supplies: disposable medical instruments, appliances, and articles shall be used as much as possible. After use, double-layer medical waste bags shall be sealed. According to the disposal of infectious medical waste, reusable medical instruments shall be contained in double-layer medical waste bags, labeled and put into the tidying box for centralized delivery to the disinfection and supply center for treatment.

Medical waste shall comply with the requirements of *Regulations on Medical Waste Management* and *Measures for Medical Waste Management in Medical and Health Institutions*. Double-layer yellow medical waste collection bags shall be standardized for packaging. Another layer of yellow medical waste bags shall be put to the west contaminant ladder for recycling by personnel of temporary storage room.

Personal belongings of patients: clothes of patients are recommended to be incinerated uniformly according to medical wastes. If there are no visible contaminants, circulating steam or boiling can be used for disinfection for 30 min if reuse is required; or soak in 500 mg/L chlorine-containing disinfectant for 30 min, and then clean according to the routine process; or directly put into a washing machine after being filled in a water-soluble packaging bag, and simultaneously wash and disinfect for 30 min, and keep the available chlorine content of 500 mg/L. Other personal belongings can be irradiated with ultraviolet ray for 1 h or moisture-resistant articles can be soaked in disinfectant for 30 min.

Corpse handling: after the patient dies, the movement and handling of the corpse shall be minimized, and the corpse shall be handled in a timely manner by trained staff under strict protection. Use 3000–5000 mg/L chlorine-containing disinfectant cotton ball or gauze to fill all open channels or wounds of the patient's mouth, nose, ear, anus, tracheotomy, etc. Wrap the corpse in a double-layer cloth soaked with disinfectant and put it into a double-layer corpse bag. The civil affairs department will send a special vehicle directly to the designated place for cremation as soon as possible.

2.2 Staff Management

Li Jiang, Qian Liu and Yunzhou Fan

2.2.1 Work Discipline of Medical Staff

In order to strengthen the prevention and control of COVID-19 infection in the hospital and prevent cross-infection among hospital staff, medical staff shall abide by the following work disciplines:

All staff shall truthfully report to the hospital whether they have had close contact with highly suspected or infected COVID-19 patients.

All staff shall have their body temperature monitored daily before taking up their posts and monitoring records shall be made.

Staff in each ward area shall avoid gathering for meals. The number of people eating together shall not exceed 10. The dining distance shall be kept beyond 1 m. After taking off masks, it is forbidden to talk to each other and make phone calls.

If the staffs have any discomfort symptoms, the staff shall immediately report to the person in charge of each medical team, who shall also report to the infection department and the public health department of the hospital.

Except for the on-duty staff, other staff must leave the ward area as soon as possible and are not allowed to stay in the ward area and cleaning area.

Infection prevention and control personnel of each medical team in the hospital need to strengthen supervision and training of infection prevention and control measures of this medical team and personal protective measures of medical team members, and correct problems found instantly.

2.2.2 Precautions for Medical Staff to Take Public Transportation During COVID-19

Before taking public vehicles, wear surgical masks or medical protective masks regularly, and carry out daily self-health monitoring.

Do not eat or drink when taking public vehicles.

When taking public vehicles keep the distance with others as far as possible and reduce the conversation; try to be in a single row and single seat, and reduce touching the articles in the vehicle.

When taking public vehicles, open the windows as much as possible to keep the air in the vehicle flowing.

When taking public vehicles, medical staff shall carry ABHR with them, and carry out hand hygiene in time after touching frequently contacted surfaces (such as vehicle handles and window keys).

Medical staff shall record the time and license plate number of daily public vehicle so as to carry out epidemiological investigation when necessary.

If the medical staff feel unwell, suspected, or confirmed to be infected with novel coronavirus, they need to timely and truthfully report the date, time, and license plate number of the public vehicle taken and assist in the epidemiological investigation of close contacts.

If taking online taxi-hailing service, try not to share it with many people, and choose the rear seat when taking it.

2.3 Personal Protection in Different Scenes

Li Jiang, Qian Liu and Yunzhou Fan

2.3.1 Personal Protection of Medical Staff

2.3.1.1 Personal Protective Equipment and Application

Personal protective equipment shall be used by all personnel who come into contact with or may come into contact with COVID-19 cases and infected persons, contaminants (blood, body fluids, secretions, vomitus and excrement, etc.) and their contaminated articles or environmental surfaces, including:

2.3.1.1.1 Gloves

When entering contaminated areas or carrying out diagnosis and treatment operations, wear disposable rubber or nitrile gloves according to the work content, disinfect in time when contacting different patients or gloves are damaged, and replace gloves and carry out hand hygiene.

2.3.1.1.2 Medical Protective Mask

When entering contaminated areas or carrying out diagnosis and treatment operations, medical protective masks (N95 and above) or powered air-purifying respirators shall be worn. Air tightness inspection shall be carried out before each wearing. When wearing multiple protective articles, it is ensured that the medical protective masks are finally removed.

2.3.1.1.3 Protective Face Shield or Goggles

When entering contaminated areas or carrying out diagnosis and treatment operations, if the eyes, conjunctiva, and face are at risk of being contaminated by blood, body fluids, secretions, excretions, and aerosols, protective face shields or goggles shall be worn. After each use of reusable goggles, disinfection and drying shall be carried out in time for standby.

2.3.1.1.4 Medical Disposable Protective Suit

When entering contaminated areas or carrying out diagnosis and treatment operations, personal clothes shall be replaced and work clothes (scrubs or disposable clothes) shall be worn and then medical disposable protective suit shall be worn.

2.3.1.2 Hand Hygiene

When there are no obvious contaminants, ABHR shall be used. When there are visible contaminants, hand sanitizer shall be used to wash hands under flowing water, and then ABHR shall be used.

Hand hygiene measures shall be strictly taken in daily work, especially before wearing gloves and personal protective equipment. Before sterile operation for patients, after possible contact with patients' blood, body fluids, and their contaminated articles or contaminated environmental surfaces, and in the process of removing personal protective equipment, special attention shall be paid to hand hygiene measures.

2.3.1.3 Personal Protection for Specific Groups

2.3.1.3.1 Staff in Isolation Ward Area and Staff in Medical Observation Place

It is recommended to wear work clothes, disposable work caps, disposable gloves, disposable medical protective suit, medical protective masks (N95 and above), protective face shields or goggles, work shoes or rubber boots, waterproof boot covers, etc.

2.3.1.3.2 Personnel Transferring Infected Persons

It is recommended to wear work clothes, disposable work caps, disposable gloves, disposable medical protective suit, medical protective masks (N95 and above), protective face shields or goggles, work shoes or rubber boots, waterproof boot covers, etc.

2.3.1.3.3 Personnel Handling Corpse

It is recommended to wear work clothes, disposable work caps, disposable gloves and long-sleeved padded rubber gloves, disposable medical protective suit, medical protective masks (N95 and above), protective face shields, work shoes or rubber boots, waterproof boot covers, waterproof aprons, or waterproof isolation gown, etc.

2.3.1.3.4 Personnel for Environmental Cleaning and Disinfection

It is recommended to wear work clothes, disposable work caps, disposable gloves and long-sleeved padded rubber gloves, disposable medical protective suit, medical protective masks (N95 and above), protective face shields, work shoes or rubber boots, waterproof boot covers, waterproof aprons, or waterproof isolation gown.

2.3.1.3.5 Personnel Collecting Specimens

It is recommended to wear work clothes, disposable work caps, double-layer gloves, disposable medical protective suit, medical protective masks (N95 and above), protective face shields, work shoes or rubber boots, and waterproof boot covers. When necessary, waterproof aprons or waterproof isolation gown can be worn.

2.3.1.3.6 Laboratory Staff

It is recommended to at least wear work clothes, disposable work caps, double-layer gloves, disposable medical protective suit, medical protective masks (N95 and above), protective face shields or goggles, work shoes or rubber boots, and waterproof boot covers. When necessary, waterproof aprons or waterproof isolation gown can be worn.

2.3.1.4 Precautions for Removing Protective Equipment

Contact with the contaminated surface as little as possible when removing.

Non-disposable items such as the removed protective goggles and rubber boots shall be put into a container filled with disinfectant for soaking. The remaining disposable items shall be put into yellow medical waste collection bags for centralized disposal as medical waste.

Hand disinfection shall be carried out in each step of removing protective equipment. Hand washing and hand disinfection shall be carried out again after all protective equipment has been removed.

2.3.2 Prevention and Treatment Process for Accidental Entry of Patients or Medical Staff Wearing Contaminated Protective Articles in the Clean Area

Access control systems are installed on the medical staff passage and the patient passage.

When patients are admitted to the hospital, they will be sent to the patient passage in the isolation ward area by special personnel.

Improve the education of patients, and inform the patients at the time of admission and post-admission: for your safety, please limit your activities within this ward.

Strengthen territorial management. The head nurse of the isolation ward is responsible for on-site training and assessment of medical staff who rotate into the area to work, and medical staff will take up their posts after passing the assessment.

Put up clear and eye-catching warnings at the entrances of different areas.

When patients or medical staff wearing contaminated protective articles enter the clean area:

1. Immediately direct them to return from the buffer zone to the contaminated zone.
2. Open the window and ventilate immediately.
3. When there are visible contaminants on the surface of environmental objects and ground, first use disposable absorbent materials (such as gauze, cloth) to dip 5000 mg/L chlorine-containing disinfectant to carefully remove contaminants. When there is no visible contaminant, 1000 mg/L chlorine-containing disinfectant can be used to wipe and disinfect.
4. If there are no people, ultraviolet lamp can be used to irradiate for 1 h or hydrogen peroxide air sterilizer can be used; if there is someone, mobile plasma air sterilizer can be used for air disinfection.

2.3.3 Emergency Treatment Process for Occupational Exposure of Medical Staff

During the epidemic of COVID-19, if medical staff are exposed to occupational hazards in the contaminated area of the isolation ward, they should go to the nearest location where there are hand hygiene facilities of flowing water to carry out emergency treatment on the exposed areas, and take off protective articles at the designated locations according to the process, and then carry out further exposure treatment in the clean area and report to the superior.

When the skin is contaminated by contaminants, the contaminants shall be removed immediately, and then 0.5% iodophor or 3% hydrogen peroxide disinfectant shall be dipped in disposable absorbent material to wipe and disinfect for more than 3 min, and then clear water is used to clean.

When mucosa of eyes is contaminated by contaminants, a large amount of normal saline or 0.05% iodophor shall be used for flushing and disinfection.

Immediately after occupational exposure of sharp instruments such as needle prick injuries, gently squeeze the blood from the proximal end to the distal end of the wound as far as possible, rinse with soap solution and flowing water, and then disinfect with 75% alcohol or 0.5% iodophor, and cover up the wound.

After respiratory tract exposure, gargle with a large amount of normal saline or hydrogen peroxide, and assess whether medical observation is needed according to the exposure. Those needing medical observation are required to stay at home for 14 days. If respiratory tract symptoms occur during observation, go to a fever clinic immediately.

Occupational exposure can be prevented by taking appropriate antiviral drugs under the guidance of physicians of the infection department.

2.4 Biosafety Management

Li Jiang, Qian Liu and Yunzhou Fan

2.4.1 Infection Prevention and Control for Novel Coronavirus Specimen Collection and Transportation [1–3]

2.4.1.1 Protection of Sampling Personnel

Wear disposable work caps, medical protective masks (N95 and above) or powered air-purifying respirators, protective face shields, protective inner clothes or work clothes (white coats), disposable medical protective suit, disposable latex gloves (2 pairs), work shoes, and waterproof boot covers.

2.4.1.2 Requirements for Sampling Rooms in Fever Clinic

1. Special sampling rooms shall be set up instead of bedside sampling.
2. The sampling room shall be equipped with air disinfection devices such as ultraviolet ray/air disinfecting machine.
3. During sampling, the number of personnel shall be minimized in the collection room except the sampling personnel and the patient to be sampled.
4. After sampling, air and object surface disinfection shall be carried out before sampling for the next patient.
5. Personnel carrying out cleaning and disinfection shall also make personal protection.

2.4.1.3 Placement of Specimens

1. All specimens shall be placed in a suitable size of sample collection tube with spiral cover, gasket, and freeze resistance, and fastened.
2. Put the sealed specimen into biosafety sample bags, one specimen in each bag.
3. Spray the biosafety sample bag with 75% alcohol and then place it in the designated place.

2.4.1.4 Occupational Protection of Specimen Transporting Personnel

1. Wear disposable work caps, protective face shields or goggles (anti-fog type), medical protective mask (N95 and above), protective inner clothes or work clothes, disposable anti-infiltration isolation gown/disposable protective suit (as the case may be), disposable latex gloves (double-layer), and disposable shoe covers if necessary.
2. Carry hand sanitizer at all times.

2.4.1.5 Specimen Transportation

1. Specimen transporting personnel shall follow a fixed route and a designated elevator to collect and transport specimens at a designated place.
2. Hand hygiene shall be carried out after each biosafety sample bag is put into the transporting container.
3. Transporting containers shall be sealed and have biohazard identification.
4. After transporting the specimen, the transporting container shall be disinfected and can be soaked with 1000 mg/L chlorine-containing disinfectant for 30 min for disinfection.
5. Designated specimen transporting elevators shall be disinfected daily. Chlorine-containing disinfectant can be used to wipe the cart bottom and cart surface for 30 min, and then the air supply system shall be turned on for 1 h before use of the elevators.

2.5 Patient Transfer

Yan Jin and Fanjun Cheng

When a non-designated medical institution finds a confirmed or suspected COVID-19 patient, a report is necessary to the local health administrative department. The patient shall be transferred to the isolation treatment place or the isolation ward of the designated hospital according to the classification. For medical institutions with isolation wards, the clinic will receive the patient and send them to isolation wards. There are two major types of patient transfer: inter-hospital transfer, from clinic or ward of general medical institutions and clinic or ward of designated hospitals of fever clinic to designated hospitals for critical cases because of critical illness, and in-hospital transfer, from designated hospitals and/or critical case treatment hospitals to places other than the ward area for workup or treatment. Transfer elements include transfer-involved staff, patients, and transfer tools. Commonly used transfer tools include emergency ambulances, transfer rollaway beds, and wheelchairs.

2.5.1 Inter-hospital Transfer, i.e., Transfer Between Medical Institutions

The health administrative department, the first-aid center, the out-transferring organization, and the transfer-in organization jointly set up a transfer working team. Members of the team shall fully understand the patient's condition.

Determine the transfer time and route.

Prepare transfer vehicles and on-board equipment.

Configure special vehicles and equipment, and set up special parking and decontamination areas. Negative pressure isolation cabin or negative pressure ambulance shall be used for transfer as much as possible [4]. When transferring severe cases, the vehicle shall be equipped with necessary life support equipment.

The cab is strictly sealed and isolated from the carriage, and the vehicle is equipped with placement area for contaminated articles, protective articles, disinfectant, and ABHR.

Preparation of transfer staff.

Medical staff shall implement the Level 3 protection standard [5]. Drivers shall implement the Level 2 protection standard.

After transferring COVID-19 patients, replace the full set of protective articles in time.

Patient preparation. Communicate with patients in advance and make preparations for their psychology and personal belongings. When multiple patients are transferred, arrange the sequence of transfer.

2.5.1.1 Transfer Workflow [6]

The staff receive the transfer order → wear protective articles → drive to the corresponding medical institutions according to the order → hand over the patient at the designated place → guide the patient to wear surgical masks → place the patient in an ambulance → give symptomatic treatment according to the patient's condition → transfer the patient to the receiving medical institution and hand over → the transfer vehicle and the staff return to the working place →the staff and the vehicle are disinfected → the staff and the vehicle are on a standby.

2.5.2 In-hospital Transfer

From the fever clinic to the isolation ward, the transfer mode and details are determined according to the patient's condition.

Determine the receiving and treatment area and time in advance.

Mild cases and ordinary patients arrive at the receiving and treatment area according to the designated route under the guidance of hospital staff.

For severe and critical patients, the transfer will be started after the patient's condition is evaluated by both the transfer-out department and the transfer-in department.

The transfer-out department and the receiving department shall agree in advance on the transfer time and the in-hospital route.

The receiving department shall prepare for receiving and treatment according to the patient's condition and provide adequate corresponding treatment equipment and medicine.

Preparation of transfer-out department for transfer objects:

For high-risk patients, choose and prepare necessary vital sign monitoring and supporting equipment, rebreathing bags, 5 L portable oxygen cylinder, portable ventilator, multifunctional ECG monitor, oxygen saturation monitor, and other equipment related to illness, as well as prepare first-aid kit when necessary.

Preparation of transfer elevator: the transfer-out department shall contact the elevator operator in advance to ensure the use of the special elevator.

The transfer-out department shall determine the transfer personnel and specify the division of labor.

Patient preparation: reevaluate the condition before departure, and check various pipelines to ensure proper fixation and functional status.

After the above preparations have been confirmed in place, the transfer will begin.

Transfer personnel and patients shall follow the established route.

Observation of disease condition and handling of emergencies shall be carried out during transfer.

Arrival of transfer: after properly arranging the patient, both parties jointly evaluate the patient, and hand over the patient's condition and accompanying materials before the transfer personnel return to the department.

2.5.3 Patients Who Need to Be Transferred in Hospital Due to Special Examinations

Those that need CT workup during their stay in hospital:

The CT application is issued by the doctor in charge, and the nurse is responsible for contacting the CT room.

The CT room arranges the examination time of patients in hospital as a whole according to the reservation status in hospital and notifies the patient's department.

The nurse informs the accompanying staff and the patient is guided and assisted by the accompanying staff to the CT room.

After the examination, the accompanying staff sends the patient back to the department where the patient is located for handover with the nurse.

Those that need emergency interventional operation:

If confirmed and suspected patients in the fever clinic are determined that emergency interventional operation is required, the fever clinic shall immediately report to the medical department, and the intervention department shall prepare for receiving.

The patient is accompanied by the receiving doctors and nurses, and transported to the interventional operating room through special passages and elevators.

The patient is introduced into the isolation operation room by the staff in the interventional operating room.

For patients who need to be admitted to corresponding specialized wards after surgery, the staff shall refer to the regulations for transferring severe and critical patients.

For those requiring emergency operation during hospital stay, the disposal process shall be implemented according to the regulations for transferring patients undergoing emergency interventional operation.

Transfer under other special circumstances. During the treatment of COVID-19 patients, in order to minimize the possibility of nosocomial infection during patient transfer, we try to establish a transfer route with less distance and shorter time for medical staff and patients.

Abandon the conventional ultrasound examination. Ultrasound examination instruments shall be placed at fixed points in isolation ward areas and fever clinics, and bedside portable ultrasound equipment shall be fully used to reduce patient flow.

In the fever clinic, a mobile CT cabin is arranged at a fixed point, so that patients in the fever clinic can enter the examination area after walking out of the treatment area, thus reducing the walking distance.

Enrich the logistics transfer channel staff to provide support for safe and convenient transfer.

2.6 Digital Support for Epidemic Prevention and Control

Yong Gao

2.6.1 Vigorously Carry out Internet Diagnosis and Treatment to Deal with the Epidemic

Online diagnosis and treatment: Online medical treatment has played an important role in the epidemic (online clinic service, fever consultation, offline drug distribution, etc.). On January 24, online fever consultation was added to the online consultation in Wuhan Union Hospital of China. The consultation case number has reached more than 70,000. On one hand, during the epidemic prevention and control period, all kinds of medical treatment groups have huge urgent medical needs, such as consultation, chronic diseases, and other non-emergency medical needs, which can be relieved through online hospitals. On the other hand, diagnosis and treatment through the Internet can significantly reduce the flow of people in hospitals and reduce the risk of cross-infection of patients. There are two obvious trends in Internet medical treatment. First, as an emergency measure in a special period, online clinic service has become the first choice for various hospitals. Hospitals are accelerating online services and user habits are gradually forming. Competent departments including the National Health Commission and the National Healthcare Security Administration also recognize the value of Internet hospitals and have incorporated online diagnosis and treatment items into medical insurance. Second, in the medium and long term, in addition to fever consultation, there is also a demand for many routine chronic disease consultations. Hospital Internet online processes will merge with offline processes. After the epidemic, users' experience of Internet consultation will be further enhanced and the connection between online and offline will be promoted. In the future, there will be a trend to build Internet hospitals by hospitals above Grade II nationwide after the epidemic. More online diagnosis and treatment items will also be included in medical insurance.

Internet hospitals provide services such as appointment registration, inquiry, and follow-up after diagnosis and subsequent visit. For patients who must go to the hospital, necessary guidance such as treatment process, transportation, parking, arrival time, protective measures, triage information, and indoor navigation will be intelligently provided, and comprehensive data collection of patients will be completed online in advance to improve diagnosis and treatment efficiency and reduce the hospital stay time.

The clinic electronic information system will promote paperless examination, appointment, and prescription, guide patients to make full use of online payment, and reduce the risk of cross-infection caused by handling paper documents.

2.6.2 Reduce Work Intensity and Infection Risk of Medical Staff

Online consultation enables doctors to provide the best solution for various medical needs without visiting the clinic.

Smart terminals such as smart phones can be used to realize mobile ward rounds and remote ward rounds, reduce unnecessary exposure risks of medical staff, reduce doctors' work intensity, and save protective materials.

2.6.3 Teleconference, Consultation, and Training System

Informatization helps to construct the intelligent remote training, conference, consultation, and disease discussion platform. Traditional disease discussions, meetings, and training need people to be gathered. It is necessary to improve the level of understanding and diagnosis and treatment capability through centralized study, discussion, and warning. However, the high contagiousness of COVID-19 requires that large-scale gathering shall be avoided as much as possible in the hospital. How can this contradiction be solved? The West Campus of Wuhan Union Hospital of China actively coordinates information providers such as Huawei, China Unicom, and XY Link to open 21 sets of remote information terminals in the hospital to realize interconnection and intercommunication among all departments, different manufacturers, and various conference rooms. It not only enables medical teams to communicate with headquarters thousands of miles away and obtain strong technical support, but also realizes simultaneous case discussion and training in different spaces of the whole hospital, including departments, residence, and home, greatly improving the participation effect of various training and discussions.

References

1. General Office of National Health Commission of the PRC. COVID-19 Prevention and control plan (Version 6). http://www.nhc.gov.cn/jkj/s3577/202003/4856d5b0458141fa9f376853224d41d7.shtml
2. Chinese Center for Disease Control and Prevention. Technical Guidelines for Laboratory Testing of COVID-19. http://www.chinacdc.cn/jkzt/crb/zl/szkb_11803/jszl_11815/202003/t20200309_214241.html
3. Chinese Center for Disease Control and Prevention. Guidelines for personal protection of specific populations. http://www.chinacdc.cn/jkzt/crb/zl/szkb_11803/jszl_11815/202003/t20200309_214241.html
4. General Office of the State Council of the PRC. Opinions on strengthening the safety protection of infectious disease prevention and control personnel. Capital J Pub Health. 2015;9(2):49–50.
5. Li LY, Gong YX, Zhang LB, et al. Regulation for prevention and control of healthcare associated infection of airborne transmission disease in healthcare facilities WS/T511-2016. Chin J Infect Control. 2017;16(5):490–2. http://www.gov.cn/zhengce/zhengceku/2020-01/29/content_5472894.htm
6. General Office of National Health Commission of the PRC. Work programme for the transport of pneumonia cases with novel coronavirus infections (Trial) [EB/OL]. (2020-01-27) [2020-01-28]. http://www.gov.cn/zhengce/zhengceku/2020-01/29/content_5472894.htm

COVID-19 Diagnosis

3

Hui Xing, Lian Yang, Mingxing Xie, Jing Wang, Yadan Wang, Fanjun Cheng, Yu Hu, and Weimin Xiao

Contents

The corresponding author of Sects. 3.1 and 3.2 is Hui Xing, Email: xhxytt080@sina.com;
The corresponding author of Sect. 3.3 is Lian Yang, Email: yanglian@hust.edu.cn;
The corresponding author of Sect. 3.4 is MingxingXie, Email: xiemx64@126.com;
The corresponding author of Sect. 3.5 is Yadan Wang, Email: yadan_wang@hust.edu.cn;
The corresponding author of Sect. 3.6 is Weimin Xiao, Email: xiaoweimin199968@163.com;
The corresponding author of Sect. 3.7 is Fanjun Cheng, Email: chengfanjun001@sina.com;

H. Xing (✉)
Department of Clinical Laboratory, Union Hospital, Tongji Medical College, Huazhong University of Science and Technology, Wuhan, China

L. Yang
Department of Radiology, Union Hospital, Tongji Medical College, Huazhong University of Science and Technology, Wuhan, China
e-mail: yanglian@hust.edu.cn

M. Xie · J. Wang
Department of Ultrasound, Union Hospital, Tongji Medical College, Huazhong University of Science and Technology, Wuhan, China
e-mail: jingwang2004@hust.edu.cn

Y. Wang · Y. Hu
Institute of Hematology, Union Hospital, Tongji Medical College, Huazhong University of Science and Technology, Wuhan, China
e-mail: yadan_wang@hust.edu.cn

F. Cheng
Department of Internal Medicine, Union Hospital, Tongji Medical College of Huazhong University of Science and Technology, Wuhan, China

W. Xiao
Department of Anesthesiology, Union Hospital, Tongji Medical College, Huazhong University of Science and Technology, Wuhan, China

F. Cheng, Y. Zhang (eds.), *The Clinical Diagnosis and Treatment for New Coronavirus Pneumonia*, https://doi.org/10.1007/978-981-15-5975-4_3

3.1 Laboratory Testing for SARS-CoV-2 Infection

Hui Xing

Laboratory indicators can be used as the basis for the diagnosis, treatment, judgment of treatment efficacy, and prognosis of patients infected with SARS-CoV-2. Currently, the general laboratory indicators include nucleic acid tests, serum antibody tests, immunological tests, hematological tests, and bacteriological and mycological tests. The rational use of laboratory indicators is of great significance in guiding clinical diagnosis and treatment. Meanwhile, the laboratory staff should be careful to determine biosecurity measures to avoid infection based on the operational risk level of different test items.

3.1.1 Nucleic Acid Test

3.1.1.1 Sample Collection

Nucleic Acid Test (NAT) is the gold standard for diagnosing viral pneumonia caused by SARS-CoV-2 infection. Qualified specimens are a prerequisite for NAT. Wearing personal protective equipment (PPE) is required to collect specimens from patients infected with SARS-CoV-2. Specimens shall be obtained from the upper respiratory tract (nasopharyngeal swab, nasopharyngeal extract), the lower respiratory tract (sputum from deep cough, bronchial extracts, tracheal or alveolar lavage fluid, lung tissue biopsy specimens, etc.), and from blood, feces, urine, and conjunctival secretions. If possible, specimens should be collected from both the upper and the lower respiratory tracts of each case. Specimens from the lower respiratory tract have a high positive rate of nucleic acid, so the collection should be given priority [1]. It is required to master the method and timing of specimen collection to improve the NAT sensitivity. Multiple sampling can be performed according to the patient's process or if the research requires, improving the positive rate of NAT and avoiding missing diagnosis. The combination testing on multiple specimens from the respiratory tract, feces, blood, saliva, etc. is conducive to improving the diagnostic sensitivity of suspected cases, as well as to observe the efficacy on patients and formulate reasonable isolation management measures after their discharge. If the specimens are collected in a noninvasive manner, such as from the saliva, it can reduce the patient's pain and be easily accepted by the patient [2].

3.1.1.2 Nuclei Acid Testing

In general, the real-time reverse transcription PCR (rRT-PCR) is used for NAT [3]. Proceed the NAT as directed by the kit instructions. The general procedure is: pretreat the specimens from nasopharyngeal swab, sputum, saliva, etc. for inactivation of virus, lyse the virus, and extract the nucleic acid, then use rRT-PCR to amplify 3 specific genes in the SARS-CoV-2 genome: open reading frame la/b (ORFla/b), envelope protein (E) and nucleocapsid protein (N). Results were obtained by measuring the fluorescence intensity after amplification. Criteria for NAT positive: ORF1a/b gene positive, and/or N gene and E gene positive.

3.1.2 Specific Neutralizing Antibody Test

When a pathogen infects the body, the immune system defends against it and produces specific antibodies. A positive result of specific IgM antibody test indicates current infection or recent infection, while a positive result of IgG antibody test indicates convalescence or previous infection. The combined tests of viral RNA and serology in patients infected with SARS-CoV-2 can both improve the sensitivity of diagnosis and maintain a high specificity. Serum antibody determination methods include colloidal gold immunochromatography assay (GICA), ELISA, chemiluminescent immunoassay (CLIA) and so on. The following can be taken as a basis for diagnosis: novel coronavirus-specific antibodies IgG and IgM are positive; or specific IgG antibodies changed from negative to positive; or compared with the acute stage, there is a fourfold or more increase in the recovery period [4]. GICA operation is easy to manipulate without special equipment, but the quantitative analysis is unavailable. Special equipment is required for CLIA, but the results are objective and reliable, and the quantitative results are provided. The serum antibodies test can effectively avoid the risk of a missed test in NAT.

3.1.3 Pathogen Detection in Secondary Infection

Severe COVID-19 patients are prone to bacterial and fungal infections, so attention should be paid to the clinical microbiological detection of patients with severe and critical diseases. Different testing methods are required based on different conditions, including bacterial testing, blood analysis, cerebrospinal fluid testing, secretion analysis, molecular biology testing, and so on. Elevated C-reactive protein has poor specificity for the diagnosis of secondary infection. Elevated procalcitonin levels are of great significance for clinical diagnosis of sepsis. Qualified specimens should be collected for bacterial and fungal cultures depending on the infected location. In case of the suspected fungal infection, in addition to fungal culture, G test, GM test, *Cryptococcus* antigen detection can also be performed.

3.2 Biochemical Examination

Hui Xing

Certain COVID-19 patients may have elevated alanine aminotransferase (ALT), aspartate aminotransferase (AST), lactate dehydrogenase (LDH), phosphocreatine kinase (CK), and myoglobin (Mb), suggesting that the patient has suffered with multiple organ dysfunction. Elevated troponin (cTnI) can be observed in critically ill patients, indicating a poor prognosis. Corresponding clinical strategies should be developed according to the change of biochemical indicators to improve the therapeutic effect.

Indicators reflecting body's inflammation and immune status, such as C-reactive protein, procalcitonin, ferritin, erythrocyte sedimentation, total lymphocytes and subpopulations, IL-6, and blood lactic acid, can facilitate the clinical stages judgment, which can be used as a clinical warning indicator for severe and critical cases, and provide a basis for the formulation of treatment strategies [4].

Most patients infected with SARS-CoV-2 have normal procalcitonin and significantly elevated erythrocyte sedimentation rate (ESR) and C-reactive protein. IL-6 and IL-10 expressions in severe patients are elevated significantly, and the numbers of CD8+ T lymphocytes are decreased significantly. Dynamic monitoring of IL-6, IL-10, and CD8+ T lymphocyte levels can help assess the risk of worsening conditions of COVID-19 patients [5].

At the beginning of the onset, the total peripheral blood leucocyte is normal or decreased, and the lymphocyte count is decreased. Patients with a lower absolute lymphocyte value generally have a poor prognosis, and peripheral blood lymphocytes in critical patients show a progressive decrease. Elevated Neutrophil to Lymphocyte Ratio (NLR) is an independent risk factor affecting the occurrence of severe illness [6]. Patients with SARS-CoV-2 infection may develop hypoxemia, multiple organ dysfunction, etc., leading to coagulopathy and even DIC. Close monitoring of coagulation indicators in critical patients can facilitate early intervention and reduce mortality. Certain severe patients have decreased platelet counts, prolonged prothrombin time, prolonged activated partial thromboplastin time, decreased fibrinogen concentration, and significantly elevated D-dimer and FDP levels. These are potential risk factors for poor prognosis of patients [7].

3.3 Lung Imaging

Lian Yang

3.3.1 Imaging of Lungs [8–10]

Lung imaging has great value in COVID-19 diagnosis, efficacy monitoring, and discharge assessment. CT with high resolution to the lungs is preferred. For critical patients who cannot be mobilized easily, bedside X-ray scan can be selected. Generally, a baseline lung CT scan is performed on the day of admission. If the curative effect is not satisfactory after the treatment, lung CT can be performed after 2–3 days for review. If symptoms are stable or improved after treatment, and it can be performed after 5–7 days. For critical patients, follow-up and recheck with bedside X-ray scan can be taken as needed.

3.3.1.1 CT Scan

3.3.1.1.1 Preparation Before Admission

① Reserve a CT scanner for suspected or confirmed cases; if available, prepare a separate CT scanner for suspected and confirmed cases respectively. Preference is given to movable CT scanner (if available) or the CT scanner that can lift the examination bed through the console, a separate control room (operating room) is required; if not, when disinfecting after examination, air disinfection of other computer rooms connected to the control room (operating room) is also required. ② If a central air-conditioning fresh air system is used in the examination room, adjust the air supply and exhaust to the maximum; If an ordinary central air-conditioning is used, turn off the central air-conditioning in the examination room and operation room, and turn on the standby separate air-conditioning; if no spare separate air conditioner is available, turn on the central air conditioner after examination and disinfecting. ③ In order to reduce the viral transmission, a disposable medical middle sheet is needed during the examination to isolate the equipment from patients; ④ two technicians are required, with one operating the CT scanner, and the other one enter to be in the examination room for positioning (According to the requirements of the National Center for Disease Control and Prevention, both technicians for the operation and positioning require secondary or higher protection).

3.3.1.1.2 Preparation for Patient

The patient must wear a mask and lie down in a supine position. The technician trains the patient to hold his or her breath at the end of inspiration during the examination.

3.3.1.1.3 Scope and Direction of Scanning

Scan from apex pulmonis to costophrenic angle. For severe and critical patients (who are difficult to hold their breath), the scanning can be from costophrenic angle to apex pulmonis to reduce respiratory motion artifacts caused by difficulty in holding breath in the lower lung field, so as to ensure image quality.

3.3.1.1.4 Scanning Parameters

The technician uses a low-dose chest CT protocol to scan the patient. The automatic tube voltage, selected 100–120 kV of tube voltage, smart mAs of 20–50 mAs. Collimator with 0.5–1.5 mm width. Layer thickness, and layer spacing of 1–5 mm. For severe and critical patients, a larger pitch (1.0–1.5 pitches) can be used to reduce scanning time and respiratory motion artifacts.

3.3.1.2 Keys for CT Diagnosis

3.3.1.2.1 CT Manifestations in the Early Stage

Commonly, there are multiple lesions in the bilateral lungs, and a single side is rare. The lesions are mostly observed in the periphery of the lungs or under the pleura, and are more common in the lower lungs. They are irregular and fan-shaped, and can also be flaky or nearly round. They generally do not involve the entire lung segments. The density is uneven, often limited to small patches or large ground glass opacities, in which thickened blood vessels and thick-walled bronchi are seen, with or without localized grid-like interlobular septal thickening. The consolidation range is small and limited, with air bronchial signs visible.

3.3.1.2.2 CT Manifestations in the Advanced Stage

The distributions of the lesions are increasing, and the fusion of some lesions expanding, which can involve multiple lung lobes. The density of the lesion is increased because there appear consolidations that are irregular, wedge-shaped or fan-shaped, and the boundary is unclear. Bronchial vascular bundle thickening or multifocal lung consolidation can be seen under the pleura. The lesion progresses and changes rapidly, and the morphological changes are evident in the short-term review, which can be combined with the necrosis of lung tissue to form a small cavity. There are air bronchogram, usually with no pleural effusion and mediastinal and hilar lymph node enlargement.

3.3.1.2.3 CT Manifestations in the Severe Stage

Diffuse lesions of both lungs can be seen. When most of the lungs are affected, they appear as "white lungs" and the diaphragm is elevated. The density of the lesions is uneven, and air bronchial signs and bronchiectasis are seen. The nonconsolidated area can be patchy with ground glass opacities. The interlobular pleura and bilateral pleura are commonly thickened, with certain pleural effusion, showing free effusion or local wrapping.

3.3.1.2.4 CT Manifestations in the Absorption Stage

For most patients, after isolation and treatment for about 1 week, with the gradual improvement of the patient's defense function, the scope of the lesion narrows, the lesions decreases, and the density become lighter, the lung consolidation lesion gradually disappears, the ground glass opacities can be completely absorbed, and the exudate is absorbed or organized by the body. The characteristic changes in imaging are generally later than the improvement of clinical symptoms (Figs. 3.1 and 3.2).

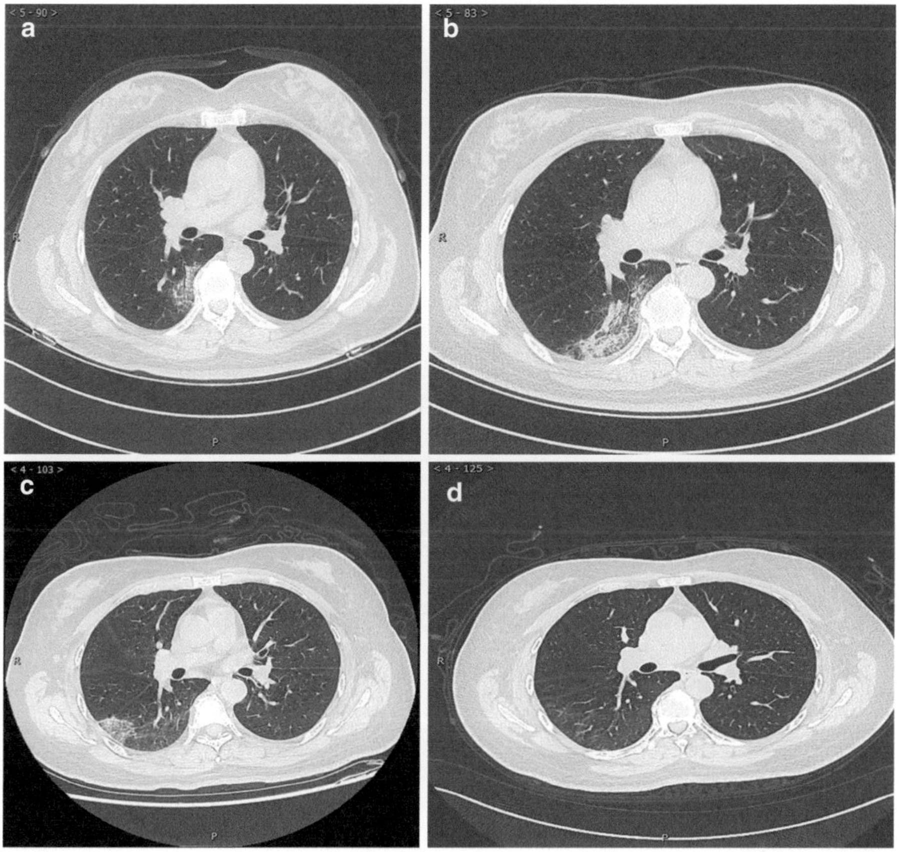

Fig. 3.1 Typical manifestations of lung CT for patients with mild COVID-19: (**a**) Ground glass opacity; (**b**) Crazy-paving sign; (**c**) Partial absorption of primary lesion with new lesions developed; (**d**) Re-examination after 1 month, the lesions are basically absorbed, with a low-density opacity (picture source F PAN, PMID: 32053470; authorized by the author)

3.3.1.3 Key for Examination and Imaging Diagnosis of Beside X-Ray

For mild patients, the early manifestation is locally ground glass opacities. Extensive ground glass opacities can appear in the advanced stage. The density is relatively low, DR is overlapping images, and the observation is limited, so a low dose is recommended for CT examination. For patients with severe and critical COVID-19, normal CT examination is unavailable due to the serious condition. Therefore, the movable bedside Chest Plain X-ray (abbreviated as chest radiography) have become the main imaging method for patients with severe and critical COVID-19. The technician should manage personal protection well: put on and take off the protective equipment and disinfect the movable imaging equipment according to the management procedure of the ward area.

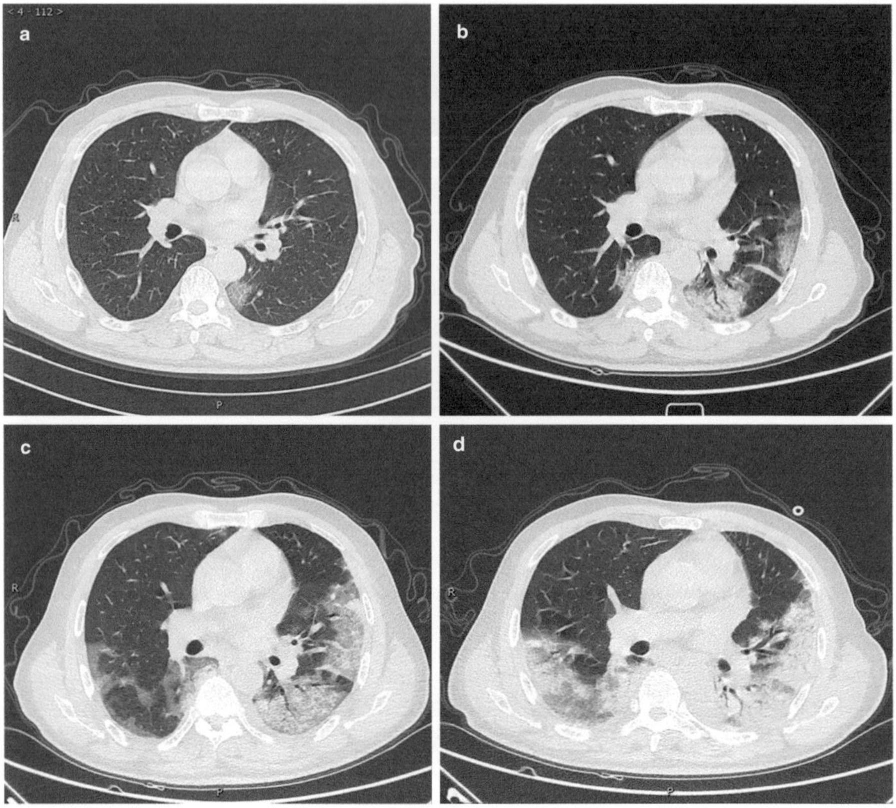

Fig. 3.2 Typical manifestations of lung CT for patients with severe COVID-19: (**a**) Ground glass opacity; (**b**) The scope of the disease is enlarged, and the crazy-paving sign combined with consolidation appears; (**c**) The range of lesions continues to expand, and the consolidation is obvious; (**d**) The range of lesions continues to expand; "white lung" can be seen

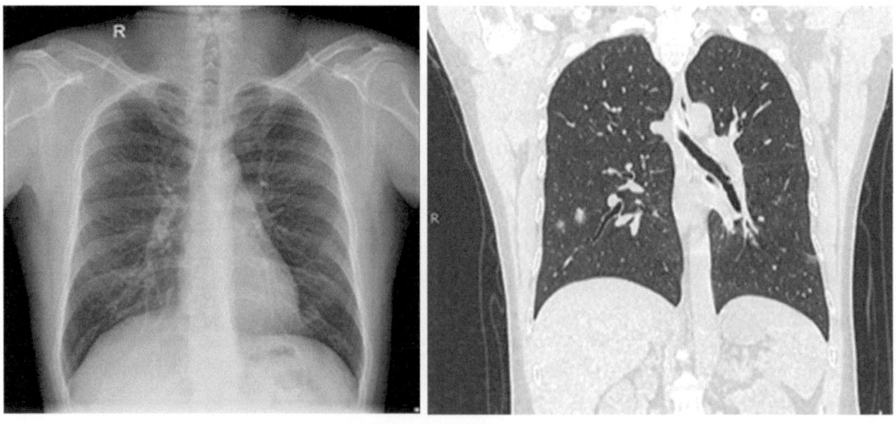

At the early stage of a mild case, DR showed no obvious lesion. CT showed multiple patchy ground glass opacities in the lower lobes of both lungs

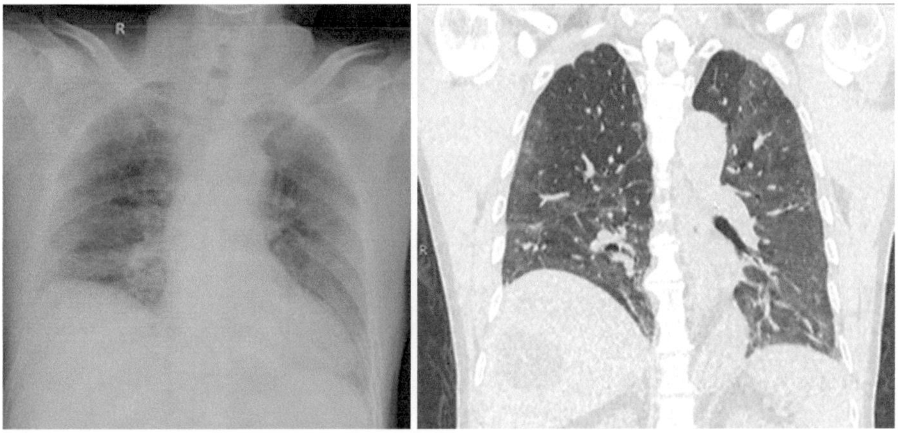

At the absorption stage of a severe case, DR vs. CT suggests the limit of DR in displaying ground glass opacities

3.3.1.4 Key Points in Imaging Diagnosis of Severe Pneumonia on Bedside X-Ray Plain Film

The imaging findings in the lungs are the same as the CT findings in severe pneumonia, including consolidation shadow, patchy shadow, reticular shadow, stripe shadow, hilar and mediastinal changes, pneumothorax, pleural effusions, pleural thickening, etc.

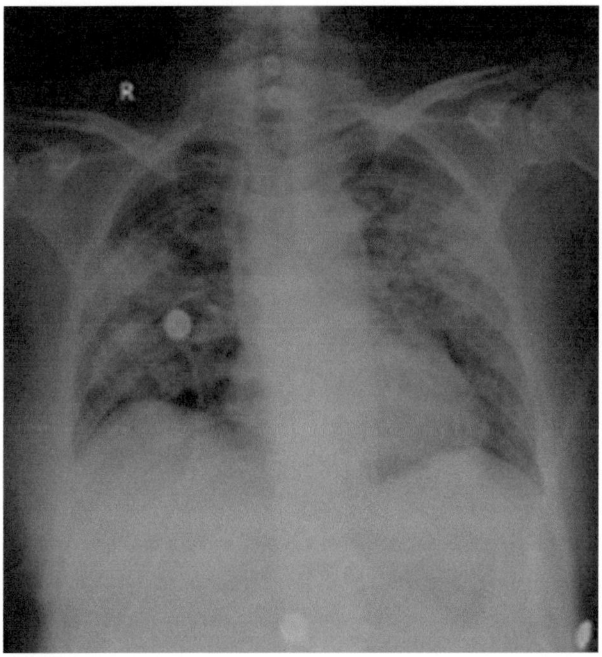

Large-scale consolidations in both lungs

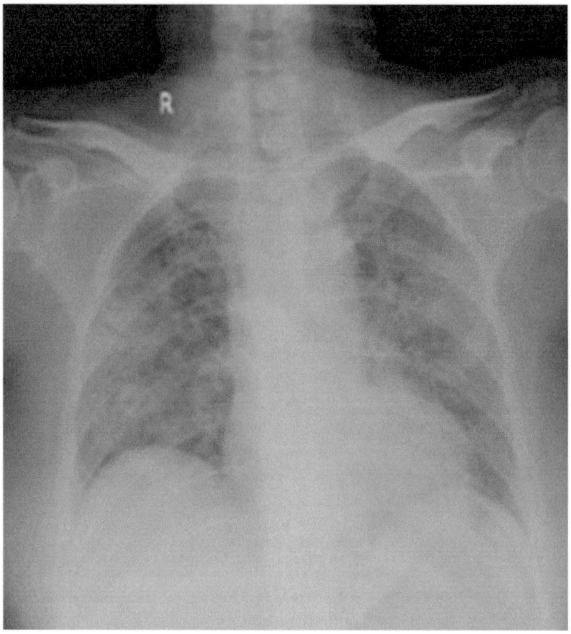

Consolidation area is reduced and patchy and renticular shadows are present, indicating the lesion is at absorption stage

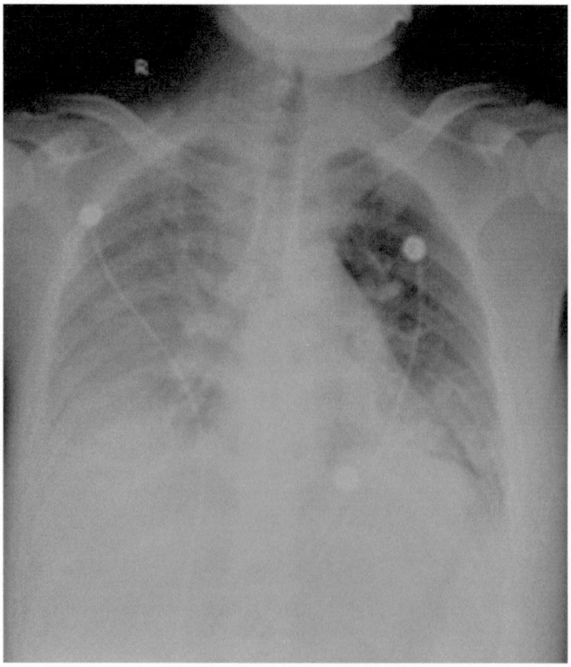

Right costophrenic angle disappeared, indicating pleural effusions

3.3.1.5 COVID-19 Pneumonia Follow-Up

Examination status, lesion area shall be recorded in the assessment. In the event of re-examination case, the lesion evolution shall be also recorded.

3.3.1.5.1 Examination Status

Including preliminary examination or re-examination.

3.3.1.5.2 Lesion Area

The number of involved lung segments and the number of significantly involved lung segments are recorded according to the method of 18-segment segmentation in lungs. The involved lung segment is defined as the lung segment involved by the lesion, regardless of the size of the lesion in it. Significantly involved lung segment is defined as the lung segment involved by the lesion, in which the lesion is at least 1/2 of the lung segment in size. The record shall be made in the manner of significantly involved lung segment/involved lung segment, for example, lesion area of 6/12 means there are 12 involved lung segments, of which significantly involved lung segments accounted for 6.

3.3.1.5.3 Evolution of Pulmonary Lesions

The evolution of pulmonary lesions evaluated using a serial chest CT scan presented different patterns with six manifestations: progression, stability, stalemate, improvement, sequelae, and complete radiological resolution.

Progression: Increased pulmonary involvement of lesions with more consolidation.

Stability: No obvious changes from previous chest CT images.

Stalemate: de novo lesions could be observed but with partial absorption of old lesions.

Improvement: Decreased pulmonary involvement with reduced density of the previous lesions.

Sequelae: Clinical recovery but with the typical CT abnormalities, such as bronchiectasis and subpleural bullae.

Complete radiological resolution: Complete absorption of lung lesions observed on chest CT scan.

3.3.1.6 Discharge Criteria

Discharge is recommended as per the following criteria: ① Lung lesions are significantly reduced in area, completely absorbed or resolved; ② Only a few fibrotic stripe shadows remained in lungs; ③ No new lesion is found. After discharge, it is recommended that patients should have a 14-day self-monitoring for health and CT re-examination timely according to the clinical needs.

3.3.2 Interventional Radiology Therapies

Interventional radiology plays an important role in the diagnosis and treatment of COVID-19 when underlying neurovascular, peripheral vascular, cardiovascular, and nonvascular and tumor diseases.

3.3.2.1 Reception and Operation Indication

(1) An interventional radiologist can use remote video and telephone for the consultation with the doctor in charge and patient, and shall contact the patient, if necessary, with level III protection; (2) The judgment of operation indications is consistent with that of non-COVID-19 patients, and the operation for general case can be delayed as much as possible according to the actual condition of patients, giving priority to the interventional operation necessary for emergency case, such as acute upper gastrointestinal hemorrhage caused by portal hypertension; (3) The principle for making operation procedures is that the interventional operation shall be performed with sufficient reference of preoperative imaging examination, such as enhanced MRI or CT examination of the operation area, and the balance between the effectiveness and short operation time shall also be kept; (4) A surgeon can communicate with patients through remote video, telephone and talk recording, or with level III protection, to obtain informed consent of the patient in the ward; if the patient is not capable of consent, the informed consent shall be obtained from his or her direct relatives; if the patient is not capable of consent and has no direct relatives, the operation shall be reported to the Medical Office for informed consent and recorded.

3.3.2.2 Patient Transportation

(1) The patient shall be transported to the interventional operating room through exclusive passage and an exclusive elevator, accompanied by his or her doctor in charge, nurse, and anesthetist. The transportation shall be completed along the shortest route without any stop to ensure the least time consuming. After putting on protective equipment, the interventional medical technician and nurse shall enter the interventional operating room through a clean passage and buffer area; (2) After arriving at the interventional operating room, the patient for local anesthesia shall wear a disposable protective cap and be given oxygen face mask; (3) Medical staff shall not enter the interventional operating room during and after the operation to ensure their personal protection.

3.3.2.3 Perioperative Preparation and Intraoperative Blood Oxygen Management

Since there is no adverse effect of COVID-19 on the coagulation function of patients and increasing the risk of interventional surgery, perioperative preparation shall be made as routine interventional preparation. For mild and severe patient, perioperative preparations shall be made for mask oxygen inhalation, ECG and blood oxygen monitoring, tracheal intubation kit, and ventilator shall be kept standby.

3.3.2.4 Protection from Patient's Secretions

All areas that may come into contact with the patient's blood, body fluids, vomitus, etc., shall be protected with disposable barrier sheet. The contamination of unprotected areas shall be recorded and targeted for postoperative disinfection (see below).

3.3.2.5 Postoperative Cleaning and Disinfection

(1) After the operation, the medical staff shall leave the operating room, enter the buffer area to successively remove the face shield, protective suit, foot coats, gloves, protective goggles and outer surgical protective mask, and discard them in the medical waste bucket. Then the hands shall be disinfected according to the "seven-step" washing method and then wear clean clothes after showering in the bathroom for half an hour. (2) The lead clothes shall be disinfected with a disinfectant paper towel, then wiped with clean water-moistened gauze and placed in a lead clothing disinfection cabinet for disinfection. (3) After the operation, disinfect object surfaces: Splash 2000–5000 mg/L effective disinfectant containing chlorine on the ground and allow to steep for 30 min before mopping the ground with clean water; wipe the surface of instrument table and operating table with 2000 mg/L effective disinfectant containing chlorine; as for the recorded unprotected area contaminated by the patient body fluid, use 5000 mg/L disinfectant containing chlorine to mop the area repeatedly. (4) After cleaning, close the operating room for at least 2 h and perform ultraviolet disinfection for an hour. (5) After disinfection, contact the infection office for object surface and air sampling. (6) All medical wastes shall be discarded into the double-layer medical waste bag and sealed for transportation. The bag shall be specially labeled with "Corona Virus Disease 2019" (referred as COVID-19) and disposed strictly as per regulations.

3.4 Ultrasonography and Treatment

Mingxing Xie and Jing Wang

Corona Virus Disease 2019, referred as "COVID-19," is characterized by rapid transmission, rapid progression, and high rate of server and critical cases [11]. Clinical imaging examination for this disease is mainly based on CT chest scan, but also ultrasound imaging examination. In this battle against COVID-19, ultrasound, as a quick and simple noninvasive imaging examination tool, plays an indispensable and important role in the diagnosis, efficacy evaluation, and follow-up observation of COVID-19 patients. The contents on ultrasound in the circulatory support treatment of COVID-19 were added in COVID-19 Diagnosis and Treatment Plan (Trial Version 7) issued by the State, with further emphasizing the important application value of ultrasound in the diagnosis and treatment of acute and severe COVID-19.

3.4.1 Ultrasonography

Because of the high contagiousness of COVID-19 and a large number of suspected and confirmed patients in affected areas, ultrasound examination for COVID-19 patients is recommended to be performed at the bedside of isolation ward area and fever clinics to reduce nosocomial infections caused by instrument transport. In addition to conventional whole-body ultrasonic Doppler method diagnostic equipment, the application of bedside portable ultrasound should be valued, and new ultrasonic examination modes such as palmtop ultrasound, robotic ultrasound, and telemedicine platform can also be used.

The ultrasound examination for COVID-19 case is focused on heart and lungs. Besides, severe patients may present with multiple organ failure. Timely and dynamic ultrasonography of important abdominal solid organs such as liver and kidney and vascular lesions is also important for comprehensive assessment of the patient's condition. The ultrasound instruments for COVID-19 cases are comprehensively equipped with multiple types of probes such as phased array, convex array, and linear array as well as various ultrasonic examination conditions for heart, abdomen, blood vessels, and superficial organs. In order to reduce the exposure time of sonographer, relevant dynamic and static image data shall be collected quickly and fully in an isolation ward area and analyzed after the sonographer leaves the infectious environment.

The main principle of emergent ultrasound examination is focused and targeted on rapid ultrasonography rather than comprehensive routine measurement.

3.4.1.1 Pulmonary and Thoracic Examination

3.4.1.1.1 Quantification and Localization of Pleural Effusion

Make qualitative and quantitative diagnosis on pleural effusion, and make identification and localization for the patients in need of catheter drainage therapy.

3.4.1.1.2 Auxiliary Diagnosis of Pneumonia

The lesions around the lungs caused by COVID-19 will increase the ultrasound penetration of pulmonary tissue. Therefore, the changes in the lungs should be determined through echo observation for lung ultrasound: including water content increases in lungs, inflammatory lesions, and severity and consolidation of inflammation. This observation method is applicable for the dynamic observation of lung lesions in the early, progression and severe stages of COVID-19, and for the determination on the effect of drug and nondrug intervention. Abnormal ultrasonographic signs of pneumonia include: disappearance of line-A and lung sliding sign, disappearance of B-line, pulmonary consolidation, air bronchogram, and localized or small amount of pleural effusion [12, 13] (Figs. 3.3 and 3.4).

3.4.1.1.3 With Pneumothorax Diagnosis for Auxiliary, Ultrasound Abnormal Signs of Pneumothorax Include

1 disappearance of lung sliding sign and appearance of "lung point."

3.4.1.1.4 Pediatric Lung Examination

Children are the vulnerable population for COVID-19 infection. The application of lung ultrasound in pediatrics is relatively mature. Normal characteristics of lung ultrasound image: same as those of adult lung ultrasound. It should be noted that

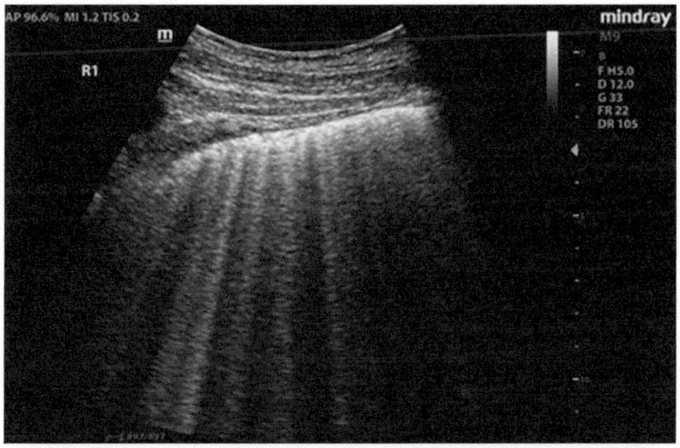

Fig. 3.3 Increases in line-B in the right thoracic cavity with rough pleural line

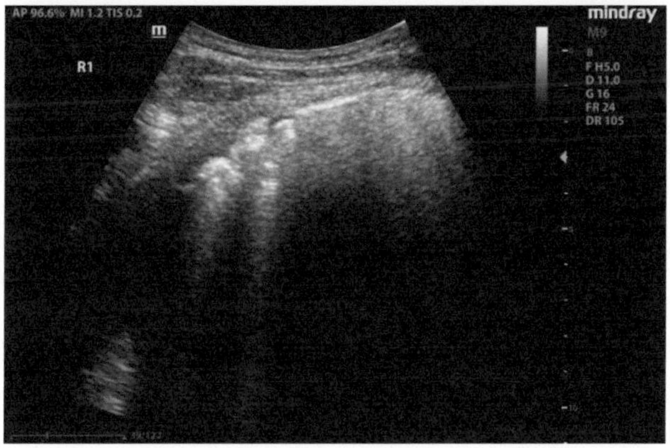

Fig. 3.4 Right lung consolidation with air bronchogram

newborn infants may develop sparse B lines in some lung fields within Days 3–7 after birth, which disappears after a few days with the infant development.

3.4.1.2 Cardiac Examination

The disease progresses rapidly in severe COVID-19 patients, and cardiac injury occurs in approximately 31% of critical patients. Bedside echocardiography in COVID-19 can timely help clinical medical decision-making via combined cardiopulmonary and vascular diagnostic assessment. For clinical heart, focused and targeted assessment of heart damage is required (Fig. 3.5).

Rapid assessment of left and right heart function: (1) Visual measurement of left heart function is recommended in patients with normal ventricular wall motion. (2) M-mode assessment of left heart function is recommended for diffuse attenuation of ventricular wall motion. (3) Abnormal regional wall motion can be assessed using the uniplanar or biplanar Simpson method. (4) The maximum systolic excursion of the tricuspid annular plane (TAPSE) is measured by visual inspection of right ventricular wall motion or M-mode method, if necessary, and the right ventricular fractional area change rate (RVFAC) is estimated by the two-dimensional method.

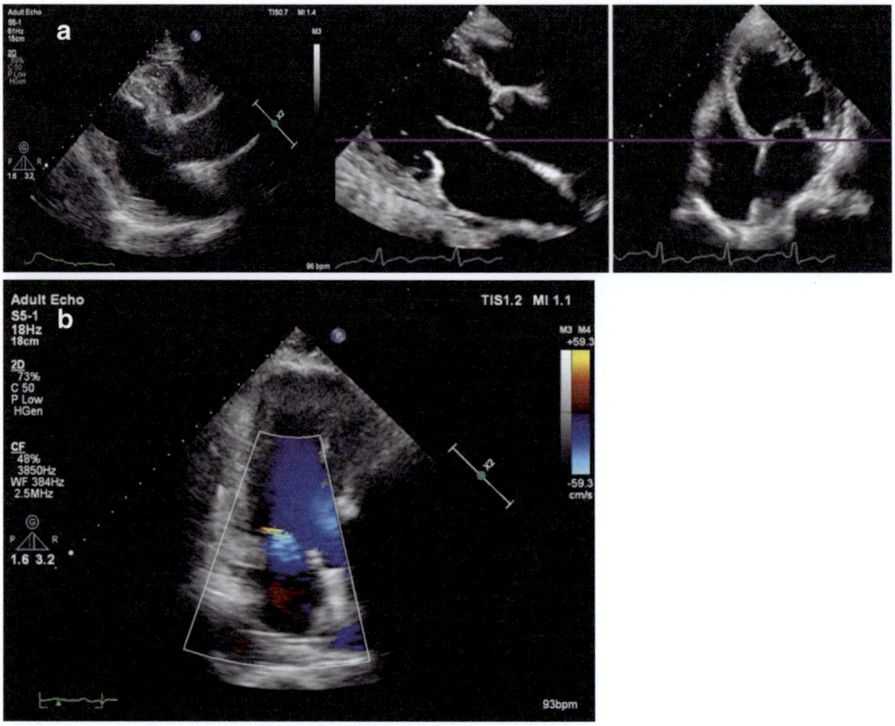

Fig. 3.5 (**a**) Left heart enlargement and reduced left heart function in patients with COVID-19 (**b**) Mitral regurgitation

Assessment of pulmonary artery pressure: Pulmonary artery pressure changes can be dynamically observed via ultrasound so as to adjust diagnostic and therapeutic strategies in a timely manner. Pulmonary artery systolic pressure is estimated using tricuspid regurgitation method or pulmonary venous reflux in the absence of right ventricular outflow tract stenosis.

Measurement of the width of the vein and its variation with respiration.

Rapid identification of pericardial effusion and localization: Observation of subxiphoid and parasternal sections is recommended.

Exclusion of other cardiac structural abnormalities, valvular heart disease, cardiomyopathy, myocardial infarction, infective endocarditis, aortic dissection, and other diseases. Comprehensive routine measurement is not necessary.

Ultrasound monitoring supported by ICU and ECMO: In ICU patients, left atrial pressure and vein width are dynamically monitored to determine whether fluid therapy shall be terminated [14, 15]. During the ECMO support, echocardiography can detect the size of the cardiac chamber, monitor whether the blood flow is emptied, and evaluate cardiac function and lung changes; ultrasound is used to determine the presence or absence of lung recruitment before weaning.

3.4.1.3 Examination for Peripheral Vascular Thrombosis

Ultrasound examination shall rule out the presence or absence of deep venous thrombosis and arterial embolism in the peripheral vessels of the extremities in the early phase, determine the distribution range of thrombosis, etc., so as to reduce the risk of systemic and pulmonary embolism, especially the increased risk of deep venous thrombosis in bedridden patients with COVID-19. Severe patients with COVID-19, especially the elderly and those with underlying diseases, may have multiple other risk factors that further increase the risk of embolism. Bedside high-frequency ultrasound has irreplaceable advantages in the detection and dynamic observation of lower extremity deep venous thrombosis in COVID-19 patients. Focused and targeted rapid examination of blood vessels shall still be emphasized during the epidemic.

3.4.1.4 Blood Volume Assessment

Volume assessment shall include assessment of volume status and volume responsiveness. The common evaluation indicators of ultrasound examination include left ventricular end-diastolic dimension (LVEDD), Left ventricular end-diastolic volume (LVEDV), and internal diameter of the inferior vein. The internal diameter of the inferior vein is narrowed in the hypovolemia patients. Under conditions of spontaneous quiet breathing, the diameter of the vein less than 9 mm indicates hypovolemia. LVEDD less than 35 mm, etc., also indicates possible volume depletion. Ultrasound indicators can be used for volume or volume responsiveness assessment, but cannot completely replace other assessment means, so a comprehensive analysis is still required.

3.4.2 Interventional Ultrasound

Interventional ultrasound examination in the isolation ward area shall be strictly performed for the relevant indications as per the standards for ultrasound interventional diagnosis and treatment. Level III protection is required.

Interventional ultrasound can be used for quantitation of serous membrane effusion and ultrasound-guided puncture localization and catheterization.

Ultrasound-guided peripheral and central venous puncture, catheterization, and other related interventional therapy. In the rescue of emergent and critical cases, venous access can be rapidly established by ultrasound-guided peripheral and central venous catheterization. Interventional ultrasound is applicable for many conditions such as difficulty in blind venous puncture, urgent need for blood sample collection or intravenous infusion; long-term central venous catheterization and thrombolysis [16].

Ultrasound-guided lower extremity venous filter placement in real time to prevent lower extremity venous thrombosis from entering into the right heart system, resulting in the risk of pulmonary embolism (Fig. 3.6).

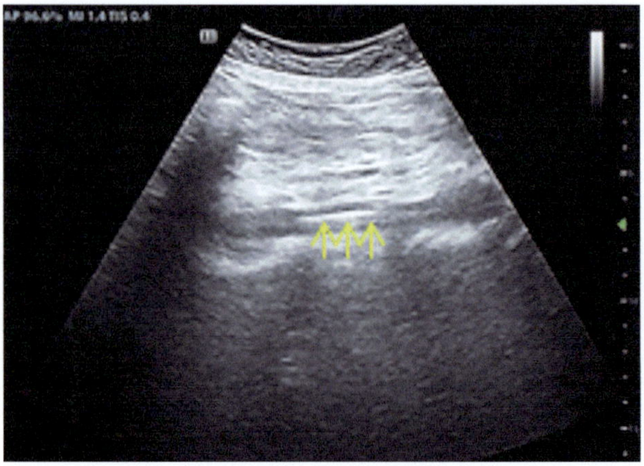

Fig. 3.6 Image after the filter released via ultrasound-guided vein filter implantation (yellow arrow shows the echo of the filter)

3.5 Primary Screening for Disseminated Intravascular Coagulation

Yadan Wang, Fanjun Cheng, and Yu Hu

3.5.1 Overview

Disseminated Intravascular Coagulation (DIC) is a clinical syndrome characterized by hemorrhage and microcirculatory failure on the basis of various diseases, in which pathogenic factors damage the microvascular system, leading to coagulation activation, systemic formation of microvascular thrombosis, massive consumption of coagulation factors, and secondary hyperfibrinolysis [17]. Multiple organ damage, inflammatory factor storm, and secondary bacterial and fungal infections in critical COVID-19 patients are most of the important factors that can induce DIC.

3.5.2 Diagnoses

The diagnosis of DIC depends on dynamic observation and comprehensive judgment of clinical pictures and laboratory parameters [17].

3.5.2.1 Clinical Characteristics

Multiple bleeding tendencies are one of the most common clinical pictures of DIC, but rarely occurs to the critical COVID-19 patients based on our observation, while microcirculatory disturbances and organ function injuries or even failure are commonly observed [18, 19]. The specific manifestations included: increased respiratory distress in a short period, abnormal liver and renal function/disturbance of consciousness, myocardial damage, and shock, which cannot be explained by other causes. The old age and various complications of COVID-19 patients, combined with the effects of therapeutic drugs, disturbing clinical judgment. Dynamic observation and careful screening are required during the diagnosis and treatment process to detect early warning signs and perform early intervention as soon as possible.

3.5.2.2 Laboratory Indicators

The sensitivity and specificity of a single indicator for the diagnosis of DIC are poor, so comprehensive analysis and dynamic observation are required. The value of laboratory parameters for the early warning on COVID-19 with DIC varies, and their sensitivities are as follows: increased D-dimer > decreased platelet > prolonged PT > decreased fibrinogen > prolonged APTT; and specificities are as follows: progressive decreases in fibrinogen > progressive decreases in platelets > prolonged APTT > increased D-dimer (the above sequences are defined as per clinical practice experiences and shall be confirmed by clinical studies).

3.5.2.2.1 D-Dimer

According to the published descriptive literature on the clinical characteristics of COVID-19 patients [20–22], the high proportion of increased D-dimer is at 36–46.4% and at 59.6% in critical patients. The D-dimer level is significantly different between ICU patients and non-ICU patients (414 mg/L vs. 166 mg/L); Progressive increase in D-dimer is an early warning sign of disease aggravation and DIC occurrence. D-dimer presents high sensitivity and low specificity for the diagnosis of DIC.

3.5.2.2.2 Platelets

Most COVID-19 patients showed with normal or with mildly increased platelet counts, sometimes with decreased ones especially in severe and deadly patients [20, 22, 23]. The absolute value of platelets is of limited value in the assessment of DIC, and a dynamic decrease in platelet count indicates the occurrence of DIC better.

3.5.2.2.3 Fibrinogen

Fibrinogen, as an acute reactive protein, can be significantly increased in mild COVID-19 patients and in the early stages of disease in severe patients [20–23] and possibly decreased in the late stages of severe patients in the presence of DIC with consumptive hypocoagulability [18, 24]. Therefore, for the diagnosis of DIC, fibrinogens have low sensitivity and high specificity. For critical patients, a progressive decrease in fibrinogen requires vigilance.

3.5.2.2.4 Prothrombin Time/Activation of Partial Thromboplastin Time

30% of COVID-19 patients exhibit a shortened prothrombin time (PT), 16% of them exhibit a shortened activation of partial thromboplastin time (APTT), while PT and APTT are prolonged only in 5 and 6% of patients [20]. At different stages of

DIC in COVID-19, PT and APTT showed different characteristics as hypercoagulability, PT and APTT are shortened or normal at early stage, and consumptive hypocoagulability at late stage, PT and APTT are prolonged with higher sensitivity in PT than APTT.

3.5.2.3 DIC Diagnosis and Scoring System and WeChat APP

In order to accurately quantify the diagnostic criteria of DIC, the Thrombosis and Hemostasis Group of Chinese Society of Hematology of the Chinese Medical Association established the Chinese DIC scoring system (CDSS) through multicenter retrospective and prospective study on large size of sample in 2014 (see Table 3.1 [16]). This system highlighted the importance of underlying diseases and

Table 3.1 Chinese DIC scoring system (CDSS)

Item	Score
Primary disease leading to DIC exists	2
Clinical picture	
Severe or multiple bleeding tendency that cannot be interpreted with primary disease	1
Microcirculatory disturbance or shock that cannot be interpreted with primary disease	1
Extensive skin, mucous embolism, focal ischemic necrosis, falling off and elcosis, functional failure of lung, kidney, brain, and other organs with cause unknown	1
Laboratory indicators	
Platelet count	
Nonmalignant blood disease	
$\geq 100 \times 10^9/L$	0
80–< $100 \times 10^9/L$	1
$<80 \times 10^9/L$	2
Decrease within 24 h ≥50%	1
Malignant blood disease	
$<50 \times 10^9/L$	1
Decrease within 24 h ≥50%	1
D-dimer	
<5 mg/L	0
5 ~ <9 mg/L	2
≥9 mg/L	3
PT and APTT extension	
PT extension <3 s and APTT extension<10 s	0
PT extension ≥3 s or APTT≥10 s	1
PT extension ≥6 s	2
Fibrinogen	
≥1.0 g/L	0
<1.0 g/L	1

Note: For patients with nonmalignant hematological diseases, DIC will be diagnosed if their scores were no less than 7; if their scores were less than 7, the scoring shall be repeated daily
For patients with malignant hematological diseases, DIC will be diagnosed if their scores are no less than 6; if their scores were less than 6, the scoring shall be repeated daily

clinical pictures, strengthened the principle of dynamic monitoring, and included simple and easy popularization of laboratory test indicators. After clinical practical examination in Union Hospital, Tongji Medical College (Wuhan), CDSS scoring system can early identify DIC and its severity as a complication in COVID-19 patients [17].

According to the CDSS, we designed a WeChat APP for mobile use (Fig. 3.7). With this simple, quick, and intelligent APP, accurate scores can be very easily obtained by simple selections according to the clinical pictures and laboratory tests, so as to perform further dynamic scoring management, historical data export, and provide a reference for management.

3.5.2.4 Prevention of DIC

The viral infections may activate the body's coagulation system, inflammatory factor storms, and secondary infections, which may cause damage to blood vessels in organs. These are high-risk factors in the formation of thrombosis (deep venous thrombosis or DIC). Literatures have been shown that the proportion of cases with increased D-dimer is 36–46.4%, and can be as high as 59.6% in critical patients with higher grade of increase [4–6]. Therefore, for critical and severe COVID-19 patients, if their D-dimer is increased with no significant bleeding tendency, or Caprini score is above intermediate risk, or Padua score is greater than 4, they can be treated with anticoagulant therapy and a prophylactic dose of low molecular weight heparin. The patients shall be closely monitored for bleeding tendency while receiving prophylaxis for venous thromboembolism and DIC.

微信扫一扫，使用小程序

Use the App by scanning with your WeChat

Fig. 3.7 DIC diagnosis and scoring system and WeChat APP

3.6 Blood Gas Analysis

Weimin Xiao

3.6.1 Concept and Definition

Blood gas analysis (BGA) aims to determine the pH, partial pressure of oxygen (PO2), partial pressure of carbon dioxide (PCO2), and electrolyte concentration in the blood, providing references for a quick judgment on the presence of respiratory dysfunction and acid–base imbalance in COVID-19 patients during practice. It is an objective laboratory indicator for assessing the severity of the disease and helps to guide the diagnosis and treatment of COVID-19 patients.

3.6.2 Personal Protections for Sampling and Testing Personnel

According to the level III prevention criteria, the personnel shall wear a medical protective mask and eye protection (such as protective goggles or face shield) and test the tightness. The wearing order is as follows: clean hands → medical protective mask → disposable cap → working clothes → working shoes → isolation gown/protective suit → protective goggles/protective face shield/medical mask with eye protection → gloves → shoe cover.

3.6.3 Sample Collection

3.6.3.1 Selection of Puncture Site

The radial artery is preferred, followed by the brachial artery (not recommended for children, especially infants), dorsalis pedis artery and femoral artery (contraindicated for newborns), and scalp artery (used for infants) [25].

3.6.3.2 Arterial Blood Sampling Procedure: Operation for Puncturing Radial Artery [26]

1. The patient shall be introduced to the knowledge about arterial blood sampling and then informed consent shall be obtained for the patient.
2. The puncture site shall be selected according to Allen's test (Allen's test), and if the test failed, try the other arm.
3. The patient is placed in supine position, the arm is extended and abducted by 20–30° on the support frame with palm up, the patient's wrist is padded by about 5–8 cm, the index finger and middle finger of the patient's nondominant hand are gently placed at the site with the strongest radial pulse, the syringe is held in the dominant hand of the sampling personnel, the needle is tilted about 45° to aim the artery for needle insertion, until flashback or the syringe is self-filled.
4. The needles are discarded into sharp boxes. Cap the syringe, roll the syringe on the palm to defoam, and mix well before delivery for testing.

5. The punctured sites should be pressed for at least 5 min or until signs of bleeding subside. Longer pressing time may be needed if the patient has hypertension, bleeding disorders, or when patient is taking anticoagulants.

3.6.4 Sample Deliveries

After the collection, the samples shall be tested with the analyzer as soon as possible. The test will be completed within 30 min at room temperature; if lactic acid test is performed, the test will be completed within 15 min. If the test cannot be completed within 30 min after blood collection, the blood sample shall be stored at 0–4 °C to avoid hemolysis by no direct contact with ice [25]. Before the delivery, the samples shall be placed into a sealed container, which shall be labeled with biological hazards. In the process of delivery for test, sample shaking shall be avoided so as to prevent hemolysis and inaccurate test values of PO2, etc. [25].

3.6.5 Computer Testing

Select the arterial blood on the blood gas analyzer, click Start, the injection needle automatically extends, remove the needle and discard the first drop of blood sample to ensure that there is no air at the tip. The tip of injection needle shall go deep into the bottom surface of blood sample as far as possible, avoiding air sucked during injection. After the completion of injection, the tube is removed, the injection needle is automatically retracted, and the syringe piston is inserted.

Input the patient information including operator number, patient name, hospitalization number, oxygen concentration, and body temperature, so as to avoid calculation error or correction error of test results [25].

Note: 1. Patient's mood and body temperature: In order to accurately reflect the patient's condition, the blood shall be sampled when the patient is rested and quiet to prevent overbreathing or breathe holding; if the body temperature is not easy to control, it is necessary to input the body temperature value for correction during the test. 2. Oxygen supply state: If the patient's oxygen administration mode changes, a stable oxygen state shall be ensured for at least 20–30 min before blood collection, and the oxygen inhalation parameters shall be input during the test to ensure the accuracy of the test results (1).

Print Test Results.

3.7 Accurate Diagnosis and Treatment of COVID-19 Pneumonia with Assist of Metagenomic Sequencing

Fanjun Cheng

Metagenomic sequencing (mNGS) [27–30] aims to directly extract the nucleic acid of all microorganisms in the infected specimen for high-throughput sequencing, obtain the species information of suspected pathogenic microorganisms through the comparison of microorganism special databases and intelligent algorithm analysis, and detect 12,593 pathogens such as bacteria, fungi, viruses, and parasites without bias. mNGS has the characteristics of comprehensive detection, high accuracy, high sensitivity, and fast identification. mNGS significantly improves the detection rate of infectious pathogens, especially for the detection of new pathogens, rare or special pathogens, and mixed infections.

As gene sequencing is one of the two methods for the diagnosis of SARS-CoV-2, mNGS can achieve rapid identification and in-depth sequence analysis of SARS-CoV-2. Viral pneumonia occurs frequently in winter and spring, so COVID-19 suspects cannot be excluded from the possibility of infection with other pathogens. In addition, according to the clinical features, mostly severe COVID-19 patients are elderly and/or with underlying disease. These patients, because of the relatively weak immunity, are easily coinfected with bacteria and/or other viruses. At the same time, these patients with long-term hospitalization are more likely infected by secondary bacterial and/or fungal. The above situations may enhance the difficulty of diagnosis and treatment, and affect the prognosis of COVID-19 patients. mNGS can simultaneously detect multiple pathogens, quickly providing the etiological evidence for differential diagnosis of suspected COVID-19 cases and coinfection or secondary infection of confirmed COVID-19 patients, and ultimately assist clinical targeted treatment.

Etiological metagenome sequencing shall be implemented by qualified institutions.

References

1. Yang Y, Yang M, Shen C, et al. Evaluating the accuracy of different respiratory specimens in the laboratory diagnosis and monitoring the viral shedding of 2019-nCoV infections. med Rxiv preprint: https://doi.org/10.1101/2020.02.11.20021493
2. To KK, Tsang OT, Chik-Yan Yip C, et al. Consistent detection of 2019 novel coronavirus in saliva [published on February 12, 2020]. Clin Infect Dis. 2020. https://academic.oup.com/cid/advance-article/doi/10.1093/cid/ciaa149/5734265
3. Real-Time RT-PCR Panel for detection 2019-Novel coronavirus. (https://www.cdc.gov/coronavirus/2019-ncov/lab/index.html).
4. National Health Commission of the People's Republic of China. COVID-19 diagnosis and treatment plan (Trial Version 7) (GWBYH [2020] No.184) [EB / OL]. [2020-03-03].
5. Liu J, Li S, Liu J, et. al. Longitudinal characteristics of lymphocyte responses and cytokine profiles in the peripheral blood of SARS-CoV-2 infected patients. medRxiv preprint: https://doi.org/10.1101/2020.02.16.20023671
6. Liu J, Liu Y, Pan X et al. Neutrophil-to-lymphocyte ratio predicts severe illness patients with 2019 novel coronavirus in the early stage. medRxiv preprint: https://doi.org/10.1101/2020.02.10.20021584
7. Tang N, Li D, Wang X, Sun Z. Abnormal coagulation parameters are associated with poor prognosis in patients with novel coronavirus pneumonia. J Thromb Haemost. 2020;18(5):1233–4. https://doi.org/10.1111/jth.14768.
8. Shi H, et al. Radiological findings from 81 patients with COVID-19 pneumonia in Wuhan, China: a descriptive study. Lancet Infect Dis. 2020;20(4):425–34.
9. World Health Organization. Clinical management of severe acute respiratory infection when novel coronavirus (nCoV) infection is suspected. Published on March 13, 2020. https://apps.who.int/iris/rest/bitstreams/1272156/retrieve.

10. Pan F, et al. Time course of lung changes on chest CT during recovery from 2019 novel coronavirus (COVID-19) pneumonia. Radiology. 2020;295(3):200370.
11. Xu Z, Shi L, Wang Y, et al. Pathological findings of NCP associated with acute respiratory distress syndrome. Lancet Respir Med. 2020;8(4):420–2. https://doi.org/10.1016/s2213-2600(20)30076-x.
12. Rouby JJ, Arbelot C, Gao Y, et al. Training for lung ultrasound score measurement in critically ill patients. Am J Respir Crit Care Med. 2018;198(3):498–01.
13. Lichtenstein DA, Meziere GA. Relevance of lung ultrasound in the diagnosis of acute respiratory failure: the BLUE protocol. Chest. 2008;134:117–25.
14. Wang G, Ji X, Xu Y, et al. Lung ultrasound: a promising tool to monitor ventilator-associated pneumonia in critically ill patients. Crit Care. 2016;20(1):320.
15. Zhang Q, Liu D, Wang X, et al. Inferior vena cava diameter and variability on longitudinal plane measured through ultrasonography from different sites: a comparison study. Zhonghua Nei Ke Za Zhi. 2014;53(11):880–3.
16. Shrestha GS. Longing for better ultrasound-guided subclavian/axillary venous cannulation. Crit Care. 2018;22(1):148.
17. Wu Y, Luo L, Niu T, et al. Evaluation of the new Chinese disseminated intravascular coagulation scoring system in critically ill patients: a multicenter prospective study. Sci Rep. 2017;7(1):9057.
18. Wang YD, Zhang SP, Wei QZ, Zhao MM, Mei H, Zhang ZL, Hu Y. COVID-19 complicated with DIC: 2 cases report and literatures review. Zhonghua Xue Ye Xue Za Zhi. 2020;41(3):245–7. https://doi.org/10.3760/cma.j.issn.0253-2727.2020.0001.
19. Mei H, Hu Y. Characteristics, causes, diagnosis and treatment of coagulation dysfunction in patients with COVID-19. Zhonghua Xue Ye Xue Za Zhi. 2020;41(3):185–91. https://doi.org/10.3760/cma.j.issn.0253-2727.2020.0002.
20. Chen N, Zhou M, Dong X, et al. Epidemiological and clinical characteristics of 99 cases of 2019 novel coronavirus pneumonia in Wuhan, China: a descriptive study. Lancet. 2020;395(10223):507–13.
21. Wang D, Hu B, Hu C, et al. Clinical characteristics of 138 hospitalized patients with 2019 novel coronavirus-infected pneumonia in Wuhan, China. JAMA. 2020;323(11):1061–9. https://doi.org/10.1001/jama.2020.1585.
22. Guan W, Ni Z, Hu Y, et al. Clinical characteristics of 2019 novel coronavirus infection in China. medRxiv preprint. https://doi.org/10.1101/2020.02.06.20020974.
23. Huang C, Wang Y, Li X, et al. Clinical features of patients infected with 2019 novel coronavirus in Wuhan, China. Lancet. 2020;395(10223):497–506.
24. Tang N, Li D, Wang X, et al. Abnormal coagulation parameters are associated with poor prognosis in patients with novel coronavirus pneumonia. J Thromb Haemost. 2020;18(4):844–7. https://doi.org/10.1111/jth.14768.
25. Dukic L, Kopcinovic LM, Dorotic A, Barsic I. Blood gas testing and related measurements: national recommendations on behalf of the Croatian Society of Medical Biochemistry and Laboratory Medicine. Biochem Med (Zagreb). 2016;26(3):318–36.
26. Hill S, Moore S. Arterial blood gas sampling: using a safety and pre-heparinised syringe. Br J Nurs. 2018;27(14):S20–6.
27. Han D, Li Z, Li R, Tan P, Zhang R, Li J. mNGS in clinical microbiology laboratories: on the road to maturity. Crit Rev Microbiol. 2019;45(5–6):668–85. https://doi.org/10.1080/1040841X.2019.1681933. Epub 2019 Nov 6
28. Chiu CY, Miller SA. Clinical metagenomics. Nat Rev Genet. 2019 Jun;20(6):341–55. https://doi.org/10.1038/s41576-019-0113-7.
29. Wilson MR, O'Donovan BD, Gelfand JM, Sample HA, et al. Chronic meningitis investigated via metagenomic next-generation sequencing. JAMA Neurol. 2018;75(8):947–55. https://doi.org/10.1001/jamaneurol.2018.0463.
30. Chen L, Liu W, Zhang Q, et al. RNA based mNGS approach identifies a novel human coronavirus from two individual pneumonia cases in 2019 Wuhan outbreak. Emerg Microbes Infect. 2020;9(1):313–9. https://doi.org/10.1080/22221751.2020.1725399. eCollection 2020

Clinical Treatment of COVID-19

4

Peng Sun, Jianchu Zhang, Fanjun Cheng, Yong Gao, Zhaohui Fu, Shi Liu, Qingtang Zhu, Yuyong Su, Xuefeng Cai, Yu Zhang, and Ying Su

P. Sun (✉)
Department of Emergency Medicine, Union Hospital, Tongji Medical College, Huazhong University of Science and Technology, Wuhan, China
e-mail: simple1111@hust.edu.cn

J. Zhang
Department of Respiratory and Critical Care Medicine, Union Hospital, Tongji Medical College, Huazhong University of Science and Technology, Wuhan, China

F. Cheng
Department of Internal Medicine, Union Hospital, Tongji Medical College of Huazhong University of Science and Technology, Wuhan, China

Y. Gao
Department of Orthopaedics, Union Hospital, Tongji Medical College, Huazhong University of Science and Technology, Wuhan, China

Z. Fu
Critical Care Medicine, Union Hospital, Tongji Medical College, Huazhong University of Science and Technology, Wuhan, China

S. Liu
Division of Gastroenterology, Union Hospital, Tongji Medical College, Huazhong University of Science and Technology, Wuhan, China

Q. Zhu
Department of Microsurgery, Orthopaedic Trauma and Hand Surgery, The First Affiliated Hospital, Sun Yat-sen University, Guangzhou, China
e-mail: zhuqingt@mail.sysu.edu.cn

Y. Su · X. Cai · Y. Zhang
Department of Pharmacy, Union Hospital, Tongji Medical College of Huazhong University of Science and Technology, Wuhan, China

Y. Su
Department of Neurology, Union Hospital, Tongji Medical College, Huazhong University of Science and Technology, Wuhan, China

F. Cheng, Y. Zhang (eds.), *The Clinical Diagnosis and Treatment for New Coronavirus Pneumonia*, https://doi.org/10.1007/978-981-15-5975-4_4

The corresponding author of Sect. 4.1 is Peng Sun, Email: simple1111@hust.edu.cn
The corresponding author of Sect. 4.2 is Jianchu Zhang, Email: zsn0928@163.com
The corresponding author of Sect. 4.3 is Fanjun Cheng, Email: chengfanjun001@sina.com
The corresponding author of Sect. 4.4 is Yong Gao, Email: docgao@163.com
The corresponding author of Sect. 4.5 is Jianchu Zhang, Email: zsn0928@163.com
The corresponding author of Sect. 4.6 is Jianchu Zhang, Email: zsn0928@163.com
The corresponding author of Sect. 4.7 is Zhaohui Fu, Email: 1334485308@qq.com
The corresponding author of Sect. 4.8 is Shi Liu, Email: 1455019296@qq.com
The corresponding author of Sect. 4.9 is Qingtang Zhu, Email: zhuqingt@mail.sysu.edu.cn
The corresponding author of Sect. 4.10 is Yu Zhang, Email: whxhzy@163.com
The corresponding author of Sect. 4.11 is Jian Luo, Email: ljwhhbcn@163.com
The corresponding author of Sect. 4.12 is Ying Su, Email: suying0110@126.com

Contents

4.1 Management of COVID-19 Patients in Fever Clinics

Peng Sun

Fever clinic provides a window for screening and treatment of infectious diseases. Management at fever clinics is of the utmost importance.

The layout of fever clinics shall strictly follow the principle of "three zones and two passages." Managing patients to track where they come from and where they go.

During the visiting, the medical institution distributes patient notifications and information forms, which are to be signed and filled out by the patient or a family member, along with the cover page of the medical record. The patient's information is then entered into a computer system by the triage nurse.

A nurse measures the patient's temperature (T), heart rate (P/HR), respiration (R), blood pressure (BP), and fingertip oxygen saturation (SaO_2).

A doctor fills in the clinic medical record in a standard way, noting related epidemiological history, underlying diseases, and any special patient status such as maternity or renal dialysis. According to the patient's BP, P, HR, RR, SaO_2, and overall condition, the severity of the disease can be quickly determined, and patients are classified for placement in different treatment areas accordingly [1].

During the initial visit, the necessary examinations, diagnosis of exclusion, biochemical parameters related to underlying diseases, and imaging of implicated organs need to be completed.

For patients paying a subsequent visit, inquire and record the examination results and main treatment plans related to the disease. Follow up on any examination items that are required as well as any changes in the condition that needs to be monitored dynamically, in order to evaluate the treatment effect.

Re-evaluate the patient's condition and classify the diagnosis according to the results of their examination, and admit the patient for treatment based on the severity of the disease. Determine whether to fill out an infectious disease card, and whether to request an epidemiological investigation by the Center for Disease Control (CDC).

Patient Triage [2, 3]:

1. Mild and moderate cases are assigned by health care workers under the corresponding government jurisdiction to either centralized isolation sites for observation, designated hospitals to receive treatment in isolation, or mobile cabin hospitals [4].

2. Severe suspected or confirmed cases are hospitalized or placed under observation. Treatment includes antivirals, anti-infective, and symptomatic support, giving equal weight to Chinese and Western approaches [5].
3. Critical suspected or confirmed cases are immediately placed under observation and treated promptly in accordance with routine rescue intervention. Patients are hospitalized once their conditions are stable. Treatment includes antivirals, anti-infective, and symptomatic support, giving equal weight to Chinese and Western medical approaches. Rehabilitation method also includes plasma therapy and ECMO support [6].
4. Regarding the transfer of patients within or between designated hospitals at different levels, utilize the designated transport tools and routes and follow the related processes.

Doctors fill out the examination and condition assessment results in the appropriate columns of the patients' information card and patients are triaged accordingly. Doctors write information about patients under observation on the observation board for turnover between shifts.

During or after the epidemic, potential sources of infection are needed to be continuously screened, including assay of COVID-19 serum IgM/IgG antibodies from discharged patients, and interpretation of the results of two COVID-19 nucleic acid and serum IgM/IgG antibody tests (at least 24 h apart). According to the discharge and release standards in the seventh version of the Diagnosis and Treatment Plan [1], patients with or without fever and those rehabilitated are classified for treatment, and then further triaged based on the items on the checklist [1, 4].

Outpatient services related to mass travel and work resumption are provided in due time. The National Security Department implements citizen health codes to establish status classifications and revise classification procedures.

The most stringent measures for the prevention and control of infectious diseases are adopted based on changes in imported and output cases. Increased control over entry and exit is being enforced, and measures and procedures are formulated for the transfer, diagnosis, and treatment of patients with fever at fever clinics.

4.2 Diagnosis and Clinical Typing

Jianchu Zhang

COVID-19 diagnostic criteria include epidemiological history (including clustered onset), clinical symptoms (fever and respiratory symptoms), pulmonary imaging, SARS-CoV-2 nucleic acid testing, and serum-specific antibodies.

4.2.1 Diagnostic Criteria

4.2.1.1 Suspected Cases

Comprehensive analysis of the following epidemiological history and clinical manifestation.

4.2.1.1.1 Epidemiological History

History of travel or residence in Wuhan or surrounding areas, or other communities with case reports, within 14 days prior to onset of illness.

History of contact with a COVID-19 infected person (positive nucleic acid testing) within 14 days prior to onset of illness.

Contact with patients with fever or respiratory symptoms from Wuhan and surrounding areas, or communities with case reports, within 14 days prior to onset of illness.

Clustered onset (two or more cases of fever and/or respiratory symptoms in 2 weeks within a small population, such as a home, office, and school).

4.2.1.1.2 Clinical Manifestation

1. Having fever and/or respiratory symptoms.
2. Having characteristic imaging of COVID-19 as described above.
3. Showing normal or decreased total white blood cell count and normal or decreased lymphocyte count in the early stages of onset.

Exhibiting any one item of epidemiological history and any two items of clinical picture; No explicit epidemiological history, but exhibiting three items of clinical picture.

4.2.1.2 Confirmed Cases

Suspected cases are those who have one of the following etiologies or serological signs:

1. Showing positive for COVID-19 nucleic acid testing by real-time fluorescent RT-PCR.
2. Showing highly homologous to known COVID strains in viral gene sequencing.
3. Result of serum testing is positive for COVID-19-specific IgM and IgG antibodies; result of serum testing for COVID-19-specific IgG antibodies changes from negative to positive, or is four or more times higher in the recovery period than in the acute phase.

Positive for SARS-CoV-2 nucleic acid is the gold standard for COVID-19 diagnosis, but false negatives do occur. Therefore, even if the nucleic acid test is negative, patients highly suspected for COVID-19 upon lung CT, can still be treated in isolation as if clinically diagnosed, and repeatedly tested for SARS-CoV-2.

4.2.2 Clinical Typing

1. Mild: Showing mild clinical symptoms, no pneumonia manifestations on imaging.
2. Moderate: Having fever and respiratory symptoms, with pneumonia manifestations on imaging.

It is recommended that patients with any one of the following factors be treated as a severe case: age ≥65 years, with underlying diseases (coronary heart disease, severe hypertension, insulin-dependent diabetes, COPD, rheumatic autoimmune disease, other infectious diseases, etc.), received immunosuppressive therapy, organ transplant, dialysis, radiotherapy or chemotherapy of active tumors, etc. [7].

3. Severe: Adults with any of the following should be treated as severe cases: respiratory rate ≥30 times/min; resting fingertip oxygen saturation ≤93%; arterial partial pressure of oxygen (PaO_2)/fraction of inspired oxygen (FiO_2) ≤300 mmHg; pulmonary imaging shows significant progression of lesions >50% within 24–48 h.
4. Critical: Anyone with one of the following conditions: respiratory failure and on mechanical ventilation; shock; ICU monitoring and treatment in combination with other organ failures.

It is recommended that COVID-19 patients who are elderly (≥75 years old) and have organ dysfunction or poorly controlled underlying diseases, be treated as critical cases.

The goal is to achieve early diagnosis, early isolation, and early treatment. In order to discover the patient early who is suffering from severe or critical illness, some clinical parameters should be dynamically monitored during diagnosis and treatment, including oxygenation index, pulmonary imaging, and the levels of plasma cytokines.

4.3 Early Warning and Treatment of Severe COVID-19 Cases

Fanjun Cheng

Preliminary observations indicate that age ≥65 years, CRP ≥ 20 mg/L, lymphocyte count ≤800/μL, eosinophil deficiency (≤100/μL), pulmonary consolidation involving internal bands, and abnormal DIC screening may be independent prognostic factors, which are warning signs of a worsening condition [8–10]. Patients with three or more conditions above should be treated as soon as possible to reduce the risk of deterioration, ultimately improve overall efficacy and reduce mortality rate.

Retrospective studies have found that elevated neutrophils and non-elevated or decreased lymphocytes, with or without an associated decrease in eosinophils, also predicts a poor prognosis in addition to indicating a concomitant bacterial infection [8].

Damage to the respiratory system, as well as cardiovascular system, liver, and kidneys is common. Important causes include ischemia, hypoxia, and pharmaceuticals in addition to viral infections [11].

It is recommended to list the elderly (≥65 years old), or patients with underlying diseases (bronchitis, COPD, coronary heart disease, severe hypertension, insulin-dependent diabetes, rheumatic autoimmune disease, other infectious diseases, tumors, etc.) or patients receiving immunosuppressive therapy, organ transplant, dialysis, and radiotherapy or chemotherapy as independent risk factors. Patients with the above conditions combined with SARS-CoV-2 infection can be admitted to intensive care.

It is recommended that COVID-19 patients of advanced age (≥75 years old), who have any organ dysfunction, or poorly controlled underlying diseases be admitted to intensive care for critical cases.

It is recommended that patients who have been sick for more than a week and who have not seen significant improvement during initial treatment should be treated as potential severe/critical cases, and be placed under enhanced clinical observation and given more frequent auxiliary examinations. If the condition is getting worse, empirical first response treatment is implemented immediately according to the standards for severe cases.

4.4 Multidisciplinary Collaborative and Personalized Therapy

Yong Gao

A multidisciplinary team (MDT) [12–15] is an important hospital management strategy to improve the quality of clinical diagnosis and treatment, and has played an important role in the treatment of critical COVID-19 patients. COVID-19 can affect multiple organs and systems in the human body. At the same time, elderly patients often suffer from several underlying comorbidities. Cases can turn severe rapidly, often involving multiple organs, resulting in failure of multiple organs, and requiring multidisciplinary assistance. In order to effectively treat severe and critical cases, and prevent mild cases from becoming severe, hospitals should establish a multidisciplinary collaborative treatment and early warning system. General hospitals take advantage of multiple departments, integrating respiratory medicine, the ICU, anesthesia, general surgery, cardiology, hematology, neurology, obstetrics and gynecology, orthopedics, endocrinology, vascular surgery, neurosurgery. Traditional Chinese Medicine, laboratories, interventional radiology, ultrasound, pharmacy, psychiatry, rehabilitation, and nursing to form a COVID-19 team of experts, and establish a complete multidisciplinary collaborative diagnosis and treatment (MDT) mechanism, conduct daily workshops, and allow doctors in isolated ward areas to participate in daily video conferences over the Internet, coordinate diagnosis and treatment, formulate scientific, systematic, and individualized treatment plans for each severe and critical patient, and provide multidisciplinary consultations as needed. At the same time, a multidisciplinary surgical team from obstetrics and gynecology, orthopedics, general surgery, neurosurgery, vascular surgery, radiological intervention, critical care medicine, anesthesia, and the OR is established to make surgical procedures more accessible and provide 24-h ensure for emergency surgery for COVID-19 patients. In order to complete treatment goals in different periods, tracheal intubation teams, pulmonary response teams, cardiac response teams, brain care teams, venous catheterization teams, VTE prevention and treatment teams, and bone-building teams are established. Attention is paid to the treatment needs of COVID-19 patients in different periods to further refine the treatment goals of different types of patients.

Ensuring the quality of MDT is the core of MDT. Discussion should rely on expertise from the various disciplines, as well as focus on key issues in diagnosis and treatment. The various opinions and suggestions of experts who understand the overall situation and have extensive experience must be combined to determine the final treatment plan.

Improving the organizational efficiency of MDT is the key to MDT. The doctor submitting an MDT application should emphasize on the difficulties with diagnosis and treatment, which helps experts to quickly clarify the purpose of the MDT and pay attention to the evolution of the disease, while also conducting a comprehensive analysis of the patient's underlying comorbidities, complications, and daily test and examination results in order to determine the direction of the disease, make early intervention, prevent disease progressing, and take measures such as antivirals, oxygen therapy, and nutritional support.

Individualized diagnosis and treatment are the outcomes of MDT. The treatment plan should be based on individual and precise strategies, and fully take into account the differences in the treatment of different individuals, different disease courses, and different types of patients.

Multidisciplinary collaborative personalized treatment provides comprehensive, standardized, individualized diagnosis, and treatment programs for COVID-19 patients. At the same time, seminars also provide a platform for all subspecialties to learn and communicate, while also creating conditions for further improving medical staff's knowledge and ability regarding diagnosis and treatment of COVID-19.

The core concept of a multidisciplinary comprehensive treatment team is actually patient centered. It is to provide timely and effective treatment plans, to make treatment more reasonable, and discussions more complete. In the event of a major public health emergency, general hospitals are temporarily converted to infectious disease hospitals. In order to ensure the success rate of treatment, a new, multiparty treatment system must be promptly built based on the original operation system to make the transition from a nonemergency state to a wartime state. In the process of accomplishing this goal, how to take full advantage of the multidisciplinary diagnostic and treatment strengths of a general hospital in order to reduce the mortality rate of patients, especially critical patients, is always the most important consideration during epidemic prevention and control.

General hospitals possess established MDT modes and teams. The inherent advantages of an organizational, and functional medical management structure based on a scientific management mode, and wartime medical service make MDT work easier to promote. During the treatment of COVID-19, MDT has played an important comprehensive treatment function. At the same time, it must be acknowledged that due to the short time frame of the diagnosis and treatment of COVID-19 patients being carried on by multidisciplinary collaboration under this special management model, patients' follow-up still needs to be further improved, and evaluation of the efficacy of MDT diagnosis and treatment plans also requires long-term experience and analysis.

4.5 Symptomatic and Supportive Treatment

Jianchu Zhang

Initial symptoms of COVID-19 include fever, cough, and fatigue. Treatment principles include antiviral therapy, general symptomatic therapy, respiratory and circulatory support, management of acute kidney injury, and renal replacement therapy [16].

Antipyretic treatment: Fever is generally controlled by physical cooling and oral rehydration. Antipyretic medicine can be used in patients with high fever. Paracetamol (acetaminophen) is recommended. Glucocorticoid is not recommended for a fever [17]. It can be cautiously used after weighing the pros and cons. When using antipyretic medicine, we should pay attention to the patient's sweating status, balancing the water and electrolytes.

Cough and expectoration: We found that most patients complained of cough but with less expectoration during managing the COVID-19 patients. Autopsy of COVID-19 found that distal airways were blocked by mucus plugs, so the use of apophlegmatisant is very important. Ambroxol hydrochloride and acetylcysteine are commonly used during practice [18]. If the patient suffers severe cough, an antitussive can be appropriately added.

Fatigue: In the early stages, fatigue is pronounced due to fever, poor appetite, and low oral intake. Proper nutritional support can be administered while paying attention to the rest.

Respiratory support: The most obvious manifestation of respiratory impairment is hypoxemia in COVID-19 patients. When hypoxemia is effectively corrected, it can significantly mitigate multiorgan damage and dysfunction due to hypoxia, and significantly improve the prognosis of disease. For related content, see Chap. 7 of Part IV.

Circulatory support: When COVID-19 turns from severe to critical, we should pay more attention to circulation problems. Patients in the critical stages of the disease are likely to suffer from shock. Tissue perfusion disorders and even multiple organ failures may occur. Early rapid fluid resuscitation can improve the prognosis of shock. We should pay more attention to fluid balance strategies, avoiding excess or insufficient fluid resuscitation. If necessary, vasoactive medicine may be considered. See the following sections for more details.

Electrolyte imbalance and nutritional support: Many patients were complicated with hypokalemia, hypocalcemia, hyponatremia, and significant weight loss during admission. Interventional methods can be taken by dietitian support or related medications.

Treatment of Acute Renal Injury and Renal Replacement Therapy: Critical patients are vulnerable to acute kidney injury. It is necessary to investigate the causes of AKI for intervention. CRRT can be considered for cases of renal failure which shows: (1) hyperkalemia; (2) acidosis; (3) pulmonary edema or excessive fluid load; and (4) multiple organ dysfunction during fluid management.

Symptomatic treatment of inflammatory cytokines storm: For the early-middle stages of cytokine storm in severe and critical patients, blood purification techniques can be used to clear inflammatory factors and block the cytokine storm, thereby reducing damage to the body caused by the inflammatory response. Low-dose, short-course glucocorticoids can be used with caution in the following cases: early intervention for severe and critical patients with a progressively deteriorating oxygenation index, or rapidly progressing pulmonary imaging with a significant increase in the affected area (review of lung CT at 48 h indicates progression of more than 50%) [19].

Broad-spectrum protease inhibitors can be considered [20]. For patients with significantly elevated IL-6 in the blood, the use of IL-6R monoclonal antibodies can be taken into account (See related sections) [21].

Deep venous thrombosis prophylaxis: Incidence of deep venous thrombosis is high in severe and critical patients. D-dimer is also an indicator of poor prognosis. After fully assessing the risk of bleeding, anticoagulation can be used as an early preventive treatment [21].

4.6 Antiviral Treatment

Jianchu Zhang

Early antiviral therapy can reduce viral replication and shorten viral clearance times, as well as reduce the incidence of severe and critical illnesses. Antiviral drugs with clearly demonstrated clinical efficacy against COVID-19 are lacking. However, there are a few that have received initial clinical validation.

Currently available drugs for clinical trial: Arbidol tablets [21, 22] (200 mg, po, q8h), or Favipiravir [19] (1600 mg, q12h on the first day, 600 mg, q12h thereafter), or Lopinavir/Ritonavir Tablets [21] (400/100 mg, po, q12h), α-interferon (5 million IU in 2 mL normal saline for inhalation, bid). If initial efficacy is poor, hydroxychloroquine sulfate (200 mg, po, q12h) or chloroquine phosphate can be used [23], (chloroquine phosphate can be used in adults aged 18–65 years. For those weighing more than 50 kg, give 500 mg, q12h; for less than 50 kg, give 500 mg, q12h for the first 2 days, then 500 mg, qd on Day 3–7).

For patients who are intolerant to Lopinavir/Ritonavir, consider giving oral Darunavir/Cobicistat (800 mg/150 mg, qd) instead. We have recently tried this clinically in a small number of patients over 70 years of age and achieved good clinical results and tolerance.

In mild/moderate cases, single-agent therapy is the main treatment. In severe/critical cases, combination therapy may be considered, such as Arbidol Tablets combined with Lopinavir/Ritonavir, or Hydroxychloroquine sulfate, or chloroquine phosphate. Lopinavir/ritonavir and hydroxychloroquine sulfate/chloroquine phosphate should be cautiously in combination due to their QT interval prolongation effects and other adverse reactions [24]. Concurrent use of three or more antiviral drugs is not recommended [21].

Course of antiviral therapy: Chloroquine phosphate for no more than 7 days; other drug regimens are generally 10 days, or until viral nucleic acid tests are negative for three or more times [21].

In addition, patients with severe and critical COVID-19 who have a positive respiratory virus test, or non-severe/critical patients with rapid disease progression, or underlying with immunosuppression, maybe also considered the use of plasma therapy during recovery stage (see relevant chapters for details).

4.7 Countering Hypoxemia

Zhaohui Fu

Hypoxemia is the most prominent feature of impaired respiratory function due to COVID-19. Timely and effective correction of hypoxemia and alleviation of secondary organ damage and dysfunction caused by respiratory distress and hypoxia are of great significance for improving patient prognosis.

4.7.1 Nasal Cannula

Oxygen therapy should be considered immediately in the following circumstances: SPO_2 <93%, respiratory distress (RR > 24 bpm). Adjust the oxygen flow to 2–5 L/min according to blood oxygen saturation (connect to a humidifier bottle).

4.7.2 Face Mask Oxygen

If the oxygen saturation with the nasal cannula therapy is still <93%, the patient is in respiratory distress, or the patient's initial SPO_2 is <85%, give oxygen by face mask (flow 5–10 L/min) to correct the hypoxia as soon as possible. If available, other forms of respiratory support such as high-flow nasal cannula can be used.

4.7.3 High-Flow Nasal Cannula

High flow nasal cannula (HFNC) is used to provide patients with a high flow of oxygen (up to 60–80 L/min) at a relatively constant concentration (21–100%), temperature (31–37 °C) intranasally. Its applications to COVID-19 are as follows:

4.7.3.1 Indications

Condition not indicated for urgent tracheal intubation; mild-to-moderate type I respiratory failure (150 mmHg ≤ P/F < 300 mmHg); mild respiratory distress (respiratory rate >24 bpm); intolerance to traditional oxygen therapy or noninvasive positive pressure ventilation or with contraindications; assistance with withdrawal of ventilator and extubation (P/F: arterial oxygen partial pressure/fractional inspired oxygen concentration).

4.7.3.2 Contraindications

Severe type I respiratory failure, ventilatory disorder (pH < 7.30); paradoxical breathing; poor airway protection, high risk of aspiration; unstable hemodynamics, requiring vasoactive drugs; inability to wear HFNC due to facial or upper respiratory surgery; severely blocked nasal cavity; HFNC intolerance.

4.7.3.3 Clinical Operation of HFNC

4.7.3.3.1 Temperature Settings

The temperature for non-tracheotomy patients is set to 31 or 34 °C, and then adjusted according to comfort and sputum viscosity. For tracheotomy patients, the temperature is set to 37 °C.

4.7.3.3.2 Flow Rate

Set initially to 35–45 L/min and titrate the inhaled oxygen concentration to maintain blood oxygen saturation above 93%. Combine with blood gas analysis to dynamically adjust the flow rate and oxygen concentration.

4.7.3.4 HFNC Withdrawal Criteria

After the primary disease is controlled, gradually reduce the HFNC parameters. If HFNC < 25 L/min and FiO_2 < 30% can be achieved, oxygen can be given by nasal cannula.

4.7.3.5 Precautions

(1) Fully communicate with the patient before placing them on the machine. Explain the purpose of treatment and obtain the patient's consent. (2) Posture: The semi-recumbent position is recommended. (3) Choose a suitable model of nasal stopper. A nasal cannula less than 50% of the inner diameter of the nostril is recommended. (4) Advise patients who breathe with an open mouth to close their mouth. If they are not able to do so, change to a face mask. (5) Avoid excessive and insufficient humidification. Observe airway secretions closely and suck sputum as needed. (6) Pay attention to water accumulation in the pipeline. (7) Carefully observe vital signs, breathing patterns, and changes in blood gas analysis during use to avoid delayed intubation. (8) Carefully adjust the tightness of the nasal stoppers. (9) Pay attention to various alarms during use and deal with them promptly.

4.7.3.6 Monitoring

After beginning HFNC therapy (within 2–4 h), the response to treatment should be closely monitored. If the following conditions persist, a different support method should be utilized: respiratory rate >35 bpm; SpO_2 < 90%; chest and abdominal paradoxical breathing; combined PCO_2 > 45 mmHg; pH < 7.35; unstable circulation and other situations.

4.7.4 Noninvasive Positive Pressure Ventilation

Common modes of noninvasive positive pressure ventilation (NPPV) include continuous positive airway pressure (CPAP) and bi-level positive pressure ventilation (BiPAP). Noninvasive positive pressure ventilation requires attention to the details of treatment when treating hypoxic respiratory failure.

4.7.4.1 Mode Selection

Because CPAP has better human–machine synchronization than BiPAP, the CPAP mode is preferred; BiPAP may be considered for patients who cannot tolerate CPAP, or have COPD.

4.7.4.2 Initial Pressure Setting

(1) Set CPAP to 5 cm H_2O FiO_2 100%, and perform an arterial blood gas analysis after 30–60 min to evaluate the ARDS severity. (2) Adjust pressure gradually until reaching 8–10 cm H_2O.

4.7.4.3 Contraindications

Excessive airway secretions or obstructed expectoration; severe infection; extreme nervousness; severe hypoxemia $PaO_2 < 45$ mmHg; severe acidosis pH < 7.20; recent upper abdominal surgery; severe obesity; upper airway mechanical obstruction. Heartbeat or breathing cessation, weak spontaneous breathing, coma; high possibility of aspiration; concomitant organ failure (hemodynamic instability, severe brain disease, gastrointestinal bleeding or perforation); trauma, surgery or malformation related to the face; uncooperative.

4.7.4.4 Precautions

(1) Communicate and discuss the process with the patient before placing them on the machine. Address concerns to improve cooperation. (2) Posture: semi-recumbent position, bed raised 30–45°. (3) Give patient water every 2 h. (4) The mask should not be worn for more than 4–6 h to avoid pressure ulcers. (5) Choose a face mask suited to the patient's face. (6) Make sure the mask is fixed in place and not too loose or tight. (7) Instruct the patient to close their mouth and breathe through their nose as much as possible. (8) If the patient's gastrointestinal bloating is obvious, consider inserting a gastric tube for gastrointestinal decompression. (9) Carefully observe vital signs, changes in breathing patterns, and blood gas analysis, to identify high-risk factors for failure, and avoid delayed intubation.

Common high-risk factors for failure of noninvasive positive pressure therapy in hypoxemic respiratory failure: shock; multiple organ failure; high APACHEII score; P/F < 147 mmHg; VTe > 9.5 mL/kg; high RR; high minute ventilation; imaging improves after NIV therapy; increased $PaCO_2$.

4.7.4.5 Withdrawal

After the patient's primary disease is controlled and the condition is stable, the following methods can be adopted: (1) Gradually reduce the pressure. (2) Gradually reduce the ventilation time (first during the day, then at night).

4.7.5 Invasive Positive Pressure Ventilation

Early tracheal intubation and invasive ventilation should be considered immediately to avoid the risk of death due to delayed intubation if the respiratory failure has still not been corrected after 2 h of HFNC or NPPV therapy; the respiratory distress is progressively getting worse; with hypoxemia, altered consciousness; become hemodynamically instable, or with elevated $PaCO_2$.

4.7.5.1 Mechanical Ventilation Mode

A/C is preferred. If the patient has strong respiration, consider the PSV + PEEP mode.

4.7.5.2 Ventilation Strategies

1. Tidal volume: Small tidal volume (4–8 mL/kg).
2. Plateau pressure: Control $P_{plat} < 30$ mm H_2O.
3. PEEP: High PEEP level (>12 cm H_2O); PEEP can be adjusted according to the resilience of the lung. There is currently no standard for setting individualized PPEP levels.
4. Ventilation with prone position: Can be implemented routinely, no less than 12 h each time.
5. Muscle relaxant drugs: Patients with severe respiratory distress and difficulty adjusting to the machine, difficulty executing low tidal volume during respiratory driving, or severe ARDS, can be considered for administration but not routinely recommended.
6. Pulmonary recruitment maneuver: It is mainly used as a remedy for patients with refractory hypoxemia and cannot be routinely applied to patients with ARDS.

4.7.5.3 Management of Artificial Airway

(1) Use a closed suction tube to drain airway secretions. (2) Aspirate sputum only as needed in order to reduce the risk of choking. (3) Avoid or reduce bedside fiberoptic bronchoscopy. (4) A tracheal tube with subglottic suction is recommended during intubation, as well as continuous negative pressure for subglottic drainage. (5) Test the balloon pressure and maintain at 25–30 cm H_2O to avoid air leakage and pressure ulcers. (6) Avoid physical therapy on the chest. (7) Carefully monitor the patient and avoid unplanned extubation. (8) Perform tracheotomies with caution.

4.7.5.4 Precautions

(1) Daily assessment to see if able to extubate; (2) checking the vital signs, blood gas, and adjusting the corresponding parameters of the ventilator; (3) observing complications related to the ventilator: pneumothorax, poor drainage, displacement of tracheal tube, etc.; (4) Pay close attention to various alarms during ventilation and deal with them in time; (5) Be cautious to prevent VAP.

4.7.5.5 Alveolar Recruitment

Alveolar recruitment may improve the heterogeneity of the lung in patients with ARDS, but can be concomitant with severe respiratory and circulatory complications. We do not recommend the routine use of alveolar recruitment. If it is necessary, first assess the expandability of the lung.

4.7.5.6 Prone Position Ventilation

Most of critical COVID-19 patients respond well to prone ventilation. Oxygenation and lung mechanics can be significantly improved in a short time. We recommend routine prone ventilation for patients with $PaO_2/FiO_2 < 150$ mmHg or serious imaging findings without contraindication. Each session should last 16 h or more. When the PaO_2/FiO_2 of a patient in the supine position for more than 4 h is still greater than 150 mmHg, use of the prone position can be suspended.

Prone ventilation may be attempted in patients awake who have not been intubated and have no significant respiratory distress, but with poor oxygenation and imaging showing consolidation in a gravity-dependent portion of the lung. Each session should last at least 4 h. Depending on the efficacy and tolerance, the prone position can be used many times a day.

4.7.5.7 Prevention of Reflux Aspiration

Gastric residual volume and gastrointestinal function should be routinely evaluated and appropriate enteral nutrition given as soon as possible. An indwelling nasoenteric tube is recommended for jejunal nutrition and a gastric tube for continuous decompression. Enteral nutrition should be discontinued prior to the patient's transport. Aspirate with a 50-mL syringe. Use a 30° semi-seated position if not contraindicated.

4.7.5.8 Management of Fluids

Excessive fluid infusion can significantly worsen hypoxemia in patients with COVID-19. In cases where the patient's circulatory perfusion is being maintained, the influx of fluid should be strictly controlled. This positively reduces pulmonary exudation and improves oxygenation.

4.7.5.9 Strategies for Prevention of Ventilator-Associated Pneumonia

The prevention and management strategy for clustered ventilator-associated pneumonia (VAP) should be strictly implemented: (1) Select the appropriate type of tracheal intubation. (2) Use tracheal intubation with subglottic suction (aspirate every 2 h with a 20-mL syringe). (3) Ensure the tube is positioned correctly at an appropriate depth and properly fixed, and avoid pulling. (4) Maintain the pressure of the airbag at 30–35 cm H_2O (1 cm H_2O = 0.098 kPa) and check every 4 h. (5) When repositioning the patient, monitor airbag pressure monitoring and remove condensate water (inline to one side using two people and pour into a covered container of chlorinated disinfectant), and dispose of secretions on the airbag. (6) Clear the patient's mouth and nose secretions.

4.7.5.10 Timing and Strategies for Ventilator Withdrawal

It is reasonable to begin to reduce sedatives and awake the patient as the PaO_2/FiO_2 is >150 mmHg. If it is allowed, the patient can be extubated as soon as possible. HFNC or NIV is used for continuous respiratory support after extubation.

Procedure for Ventilator Withdrawal and Extubation of COVID-19 Patients

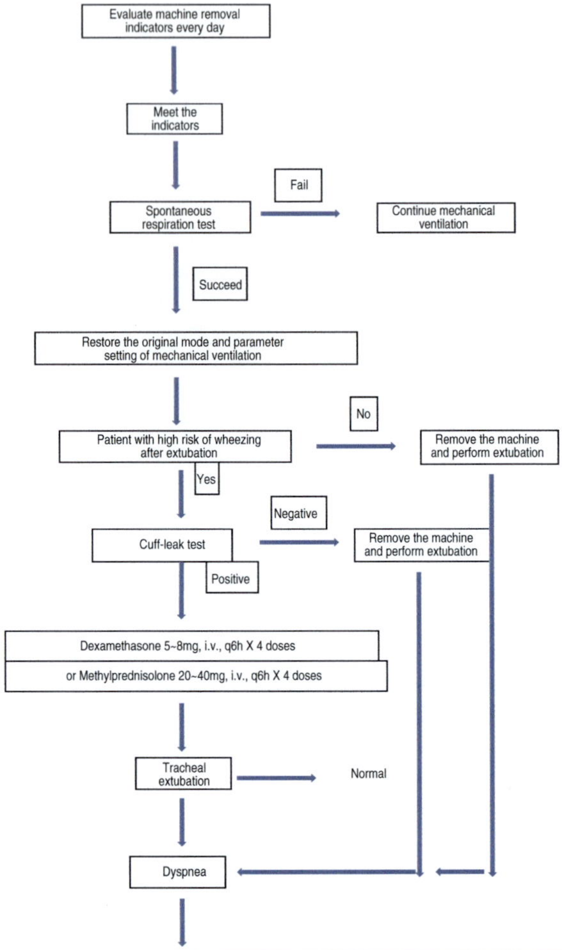

Cause	Laryngeal edema	Bronchospasm	Obstruction of airway by secretions	Vocal cord paralysis	Residual muscle relaxant
Handling	Epinephrine 0.3mg+saline 3ml, aerosol inhalation	Bronchodilator	Sputum suction, supervise expectoration, dilute sputum by nebulization, expectorate by vibration, assist in expectoration	Recurrent laryngeal nerve injured?	muscle relaxant antagonist

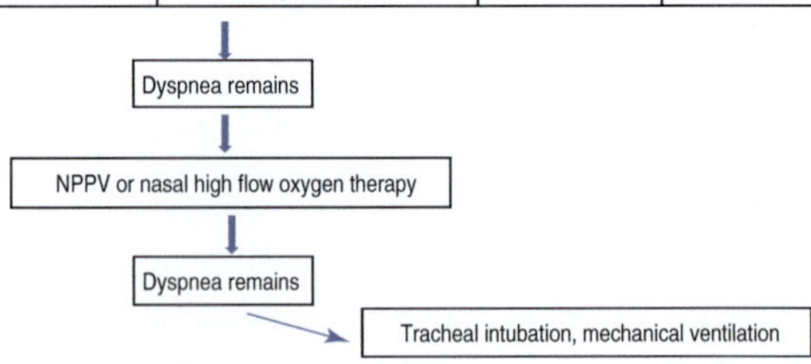

4.8 Nutritional Support and Intestinal Microbiomic Balance

Shi Liu

Common digestive symptoms in patients with COVID-19, including loss of appetite, nausea and vomiting, diarrhea, and abdominal pain, especially the high proportion of diarrhea, may be related to the viral infections involving the intestine. Antibiotics, antivirals, and other medications are also common cause of gastrointestinal symptoms. Enterovirus infection and the use of antibiotics can cause imbalances of intestinal microbiota, which may be the important mechanism involved in COVID-19 intestinal symptoms. The homeostasis of the intestinal microbiome, that is, the health and integrity of the intestinal flora, plays an important role in maintaining the well-being of the human body. The imbalances of intestinal microbiome may destroy the mucosal barrier, and cause the immune disturbances of the mucosa, or ectopic colonization of intestinal bacteria, which can induce secondary infections and aggravate systemic inflammation. Therefore, more attention should be paid to establish the therapeutic effect of intestinal microbiomic balance and enteral nutrition in COVID-19 patients.

4.8.1 Microbiotic Preparations

Microbiotic regulators include probiotics, prebiotics, and synbiotics, which can correct imbalances in the intestinal microbiome, increase the ratio of beneficial gut bacteria, repair the intestinal mucosal barrier, improve inflammation of the intestinal mucosa, and reduce bacterial translocation and secondary infections [25]. Commonly used microbiotic preparations include active bacteria such as Golden Bifid and ZhengChangSheng, and deactivated bacteria such as Mamiai and Lactéol Fort.

Microbiotic preparations can be given to patients with gastrointestinal symptoms such as diarrhea, bloating, or indigestion. Active bacterial preparations of *Bifidobacterium* and *Lactobacillus* are recommended. A mixture of multiple species and strains is ideal and should be taken for at least 2 weeks [25, 26].

For patients on antibiotics who cannot discontinue usage, fungal probiotic preparations such as *Saccharomyces boulardii*, or deactivated bacteria are advised to be used, but the efficacy requires further evaluation [27].

For patients with diarrhea, stool culture and enterovirus testing are recommended. If possible, an intestinal flora analysis can be conducted, in order to adjust utilization of antibacterial medicine and give targeted microbiotic preparations according to the patient's particular intestinal flora profile [27].

Note: Concomitant administration of probiotics and adsorbents such as activated carbon or astringents such as tannin and bismuth subcarbonate is contraindicated. Microbiotic preparations should be stored in a cool and dry place, and be taken with warm water less than 40 °C.

4.8.2 Nutritional Support

Enteral nutritional support is an important means to maintain the balance in the intestinal microbiome, and also the key to improving the high risk and poor prognosis associated with malnutrition in COVID-19 patients. All patients should be evaluated for nutritional risk and gastrointestinal function, and enteral nutrition support should be implemented as early as possible.

4.8.2.1 Enteral Nutrition

Enteral nutrition is preferred and should begin as soon as possible. It aids in restoring intestinal function, balancing intestinal microbiota, and improving intestinal mucosal barrier and intestinal immune function [28].

4.8.2.1.1 Modalities of Enteral Nutrition

Oral feeding is preferred. For patients who cannot eat independently, an indwelling nasogastric tube may be considered. For severe and critical patients with frequent acute gastrointestinal dysfunction and tracheal intubation, post-pyloric feeding is recommended with a jejunal tube [28, 29].

4.8.2.1.2 Selection of Nutrient Solution

For patients with acceptable gastrointestinal function, intact protein with high-calorie is recommended, e.g., Nutrison with fiber, Supportan, RuiDai, or RuiSu without fiber. For patients with gastrointestinal damage and poor digestive function, short peptide preparations that are predigested and directly absorbed are recommended, e.g., Peptisorb. For diabetic patients, blood glucose must be monitored, and a low-glucose nutritional solution suitable for blood glucose controlling should be selected, e.g., RuiDai [29].

4.8.2.1.3 Daily Caloric Intake

Daily dosage should be calculated according to the patient's weight and nutritional status [29, 30]. For non-cachectic patients, 25–30 kcal/kg/day is recommended. For cachectic patients, the recommended dosage is 40–50 kcal/kg/day, and the target protein amount is 1.2–2.0 g/kg/day. When administering medication via a feeding tube, dosage should be gradually increased from a small one. The drip rate on the first day is about 20 mL/h, and then gradually increased by 20 mL/h/day. The maximum drip rate is 100 mL/h. The nutrient solution should be heated moderately (about 35 °C). The semi-recumbent position is recommended during tube feeding to prevent accidental aspiration.

4.8.2.2 Parenteral Nutrition

For patients with significant intestinal failure, bloating, or other conditions that require fasting, and high risk of aspiration, temporary parenteral nutrition may be considered. Pay attention to the ratio of various nutrients in the nutrient solution such as amino acids, fat emulsion, glucose, vitamins, and trace elements. At the same time, pay attention to electrolyte and liquid balance, and then gradually transition to enteral nutrition or autonomous diet after the condition improves.

4.9 Early Respiratory Rehabilitation

Qingtang Zhu

4.9.1 Purposes of Respiratory Rehabilitation in Severe Cases

1. Alleviate respiratory difficulties.
2. Increase lung ventilation and improve hypoxemia.
3. Promote sputum evacuation and reduce sputum retention.
4. Restore patients' exercise tolerance and achieve functional independence.
5. Reduce anxiety and depression, and increase confidence in fighting diseases.
6. Avoid long-term bed rest, which causing systemic complications.

4.9.2 Principles of Respiratory Rehabilitation for Severe Patients

4.9.2.1 Safety Principle

Before rehabilitation, an evaluation should be conducted to rule out contraindications, and relevant indicators should be monitored throughout the treatment to ensure the safety of the patient. The safety of the therapist should also be ensured.

4.9.2.2 Effectiveness Principle

Through evaluation, the main problems of the patient are identified. The appropriate intervention measures are selected according to the problem, and there should be an evaluation method to evaluate the treatment effect.

4.9.2.3 Individualization Principle

The most severe patients are the elders, and may have multiple underlying conditions. Respiratory rehabilitation measures should be selected according to the patient's specific condition. Appropriate intensity, frequency, and duration of treatments as well as the monitoring and evaluation of treatment efficacy and timely feedback and correction are made to ensure maximal benefits.

4.9.3 Contraindications for Respiratory Rehabilitation of Severe Patients

1. Fraction of inspired oxygen (FiO_2) >0.6, blood oxygen saturation (SpO_2) <90%, or respiratory rate >40 breaths/min.
2. In patients with mechanically assisted ventilation, the positive end-expiratory pressure is greater than 10 cm H_2O, or there is a patient incompatibility with the ventilator or unsafe airway risk.
3. Systolic pressure >180 mmHg or <90 mmHg; or mean arterial pressure <65 mmHg or >110 mmHg.

4. Heart rate <40 bpm or >120 bpm.
5. Malignant arrhythmia or severe myocardial ischemia.
6. Recent unstable deep vein thrombosis and pulmonary embolism.
7. Coma or significant restlessness and inability to cooperate with active rehabilitation.
8. Presentation with intracranial hypertension or monitoring shows intracranial pressure >20 cm H_2O.
9. Clinical conditions such as active hemorrhage, progressive liver and kidney failure, severe acid–base imbalance or electrolyte disturbance, severe edema, or abdominal distension that may be aggravated by activity.
10. Body temperature <35 °C or >38.5 °C.

4.9.4 Respiratory Rehabilitation of Severe Patients

Routine procedure for respiratory rehabilitation of severe patients: First, rule out contraindications. Second, assess patient's dysfunction based on the patient's specific condition, generally including dyspnea, decreased ventilatory function, decreased airway clearance, and decreased exercise tolerance. Most patients may have multiple dysfunctions, but one or two are pronounced, or there may be other dysfunctions caused by underlying conditions, e.g., decreased physical activity. Next, an appropriate combination of respiratory rehabilitation treatment techniques is selected for intervention based on the patient's functional issues. The entire intervention should be monitored, so the treatment method and intensity can be adjusted or revised at any time according to the patient's clinical picture. Assessment should be carried out prior to each treatment session. At the end of each treatment, it is necessary to evaluate its efficacy and safety, as well as adjust and optimize the intervention based on the outcome.

The pre-treatment procedure is shown in Fig. 4.1.

4.9.5 Precautions During Respiratory Rehabilitation

Prior to each treatment, the patient's consciousness, vital signs, oxygen saturation, vasoactive drug use, symptoms, and extremity condition must be evaluated.

During treatment, attention must be paid to the patient's subjective symptoms, so as not to induce dyspnea, pain, or obvious strain.

If the patient shows a decrease in SaO_2 to less than 90%, or a decrease of more than 4% from the baseline (e.g., the original SaO_2 of 95% decreased to 91%), treatment should be suspended and the doctor should be informed.

If the patient's respiratory rate ≥40 breaths/min, SBP decreases to ≤90 mmHg, or SBP ≥ 180 mmHg, heart rate ≤40 bpm or ≥120 bpm, suspend treatment, observe and inform the doctor.

If the patient has poor awareness, indifference, decreased speech, uncoordinated limb movements, or restlessness, immediately stop treatment and inform the doctor.

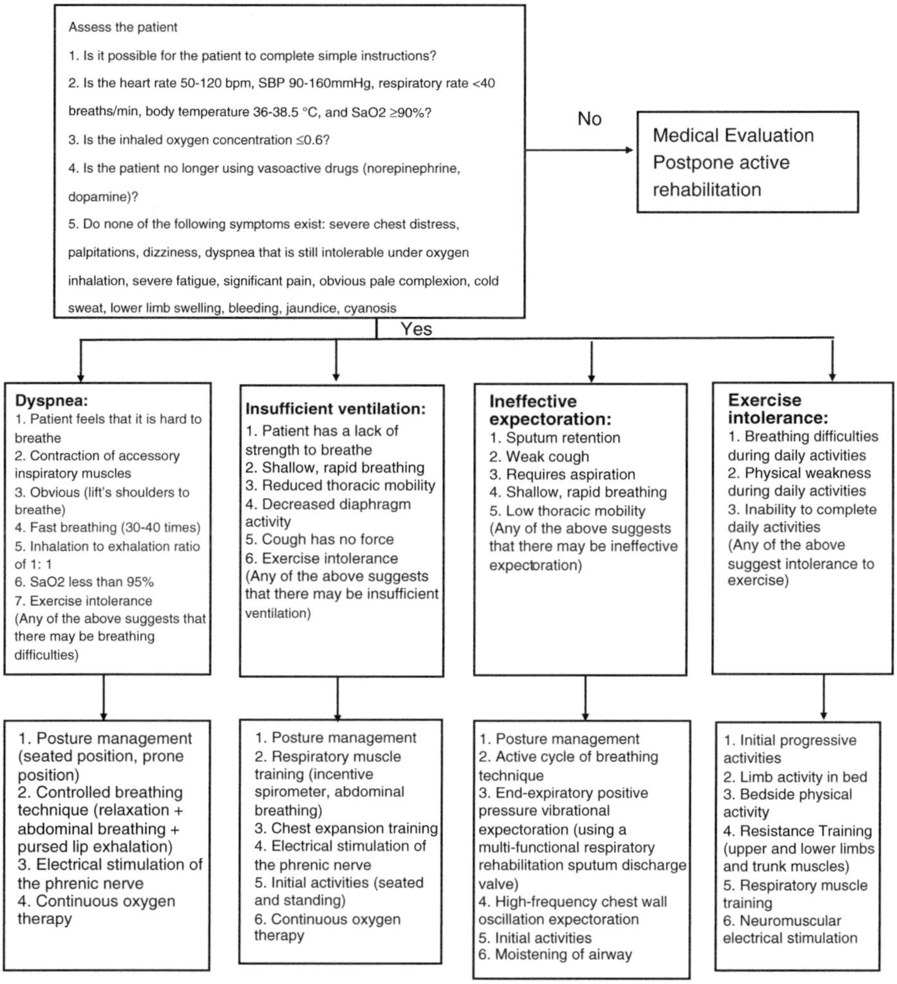

Fig. 4.1 Procedure for respiratory rehabilitation of hospitalized patients with severe COVID-19

If the patient experiences dizziness, faintness, palpitations, chest pain, chest tightness, weakness in extremities, palor, clammy skin, severe pain, vomiting, the treatment should be stopped immediately, and the doctor should be informed.

It is recommended to give oxygen throughout the treatment and monitor finger pulse oxygen saturation. Choose ECG and blood pressure monitoring according to the patient's condition.

Therapists should protect themselves and avoid direct exposure to the patient's exhaled airflow and coughed secretions.

4.9.6 Respiratory Rehabilitation Techniques

4.9.6.1 Posture Management

Improving posture helps to avoid sputum retention, as well as prevent and improve atelectasis and dyspnea. During semi-recumbent management, the patient assumes a supine position, raises the knee joint 10–15° or places a small pillow under the knee. Raising the head of the patient's bed to 30–45° allows the patient to adapt for a short period of time and gradually transition to 60°. During lateral position management, the patient turns over and changes to a side lying position with the help of the therapist. The head and back are supported with pillows. The arms lie freely and the legs are positioned as if taking a step. Change the position every 20–120 min according to the patient's vital signs and/or subjective tolerance. The forward tilt position can reduce breathing effort and relieve symptoms of dyspnea. When the patient is seated in or on the bed, keep the torso tilted forward 20–45°, and provide a small table to help the patient maintain a comfortable sitting position. The forearms are supported on the table, elbow joints flexed at 80–110°, or a pillow can be placed on the table for the patient to rest their head. If their feet do not reach the ground, support such as a low stool should be given, and the therapist or nurse should watch over them.

4.9.6.2 Controlled Breathing Techniques

Controlled breathing helps patients establish normal breathing patterns and learn how to breathe while relaxed. The patient assumes a seated, semi-seated, or side lying position, and is encouraged to relax the shoulders and upper chest. The therapist puts one hand on the patient's shoulder to prompt the patient to relax and puts the other hand on the patient's upper abdomen to enhance sensory input. The patient inhales smoothly through the nose and exhales through the mouth. The therapist gently presses inward and upward during exhalation to guide breathing. The patient breathes tidally at their own speed and depth for 1–3 min. Note that the abdomen should expand on inhalation and contract on exhalation. The shoulders should not rise during inhalation.

4.9.6.3 Chest Expansion Training

The purpose of chest expansion training is to improve thoracic mobility, increase lung capacity, and strengthen respiratory muscles. The patient is placed in a semi-recumbent position and the therapist or patient's hands are placed bilaterally on the eighth ribs. Using proprioceptive stimulation, make two breath adjustments from shallow to deep. For the third time of breathing, the patient is encouraged to take a deeper breath and hold it for 2–3 s. Exhalation should be through the mouth. During the exercise, the therapist or patient presses or vibrates the ribs with both hands. This further promotes chest expansion and increases ventilation and chest wall movement in this part of the lung. This step is done 5–10 times/min for 1–3 min. Make sure to prompt the patient to feel the air reaching the corresponding lung segment and then slowly exhale.

The patient's active thoracic expansion is also called a respiratory rehabilitation exercise. During training, you can take a sitting position or a semi-recumbent position to relax. When inhaling, both hands are raised forward or horizontally abducted at the same time, with the torso extended. Each action is repeated 10–20 times, and the exercise is done 2–3 times a day.

4.9.6.4 Respiratory Muscle Training (Using an Incentive Spirometer)

During the respiratory training with an incentive spirometer, the slight increase in inhalation resistance and sustained post-inhalation can increase the respiratory muscle strength and endurance of patients with reduced respiratory muscle function, improve atelectasis, and increase lung ventilation. The patient assumes a comfortable position, first takes 3–4 slow natural breaths, and on the fourth, exhales slowly and deeply. Then the spirometer is placed in the mouth, and the maximum inhalation is taken through the spirometer. The colored ball inside the device should be kept afloat for at least several seconds. When it can no longer be maintained, the spirometer can be removed and the patient can take several normal, relaxed breaths. The airflow with each inhalation can be observed visually and can increase the patient's desire to train. This step can be done in 5–7 sets per day, 8–10 times per set. This method of training should not continue for too long to prevent fatiguing the inspiratory muscles.

4.9.6.5 Active Cycle of Breathing Technique

This technique can effectively clear bronchial secretions and improve lung function, while not aggravating hypoxemia or airflow obstruction. This technique consists of three stages of ventilation chosen according to the patient's condition and repeated in cycles: breathing control (BC), thoracic expansion exercise (TEE), and forced expiratory technique (FET). FET entails huffing and breathing control (BC). Breathing control is a rest interval between two active parts: the patient is encouraged to relax the shoulders and upper chest. The therapist puts one hand on the patient's abdomen to enhance sensory input, and the other hand rests on the patient's shoulder, encouraging the patient to relax the upper chest and shoulders, and take tidal breaths according to their own speed and depth. In order to prevent airway spasm, breathing control must be carried out between stages.

4.9.6.6 End-Expiratory Positive Pressure Vibratory Expectoration (Using Multifunctional Respiratory Rehabilitation Sputum Discharge Valve)

The multifunctional respiratory rehabilitation sputum discharge valve is composed of three parts: a spirometer, a bacterial filter, and a nebulizer. The oscillating positive pressure generated in the airway loosens sputum to facilitate discharge. Assemble the three parts before use. Inject normal saline or nebulizer inhalation solution into the nebulizer and connect it with a high-flow oxygen breathing tube. Adjust the resistance knob of the multifunctional respiratory rehabilitation sputum discharge valve, turn it to green, and hand it to the patient. The therapist first demonstrates a strong and rapid exhalation after deep inhalation. Instruct the patient to hold the device tightly in their mouth, inhale deeply through the mouth, and then exhale strongly and quickly. If the spirometer makes a popping sound when exhaling, or if the patient feels the airflow vibrating in the oral cavity, then the technique is effective. If the patient can blow and produce a shrill sound, it indicates the airway is expanding, secretions are being cleared of the respiratory tract, and expiratory muscles are being exercised. After repeating this step 2–5 times, instruct the patient to rest or cough to expectorate the sputum. Continue the next cycle after a 1-min break. Each set should be done 10–15 times. If the patient feels the green resistance position is less strenuous, adjust the resistance valve to the blue resistance position, and finally the red resistance position. Generally, the blue resistance level suffices for sputum expectoration. The technique is performed in 2–3 sets per day, and can be divided into different periods. Except during the demonstration, the therapist should stand in a position that avoids exposure to the patient's exhaled air flow.

4.9.6.7 High-Frequency Chest Wall Oscillation System

The patient assumes a lateral position. The machine vibrates at 20–35 Hz. The therapist places the tapping head over areas of heavy sputum accumulation for about 30 s, then lifts the instrument and places it on another area, moving inferior to superior, and lateral to medial. It promotes the excretion of sputum, and can improve the blood circulation of the lungs, prevent venous stasis, relax the respiratory muscles, improve the muscle tone of the whole body, and strengthen respiratory muscles to produce a cough reflex. Patients who have a weak cough or are physically frail should be aspirated with a sputum suction device.

4.9.6.8 Active Limb Movement

Exercising the limbs in bed is suitable for severe bedridden patients. Exercises can be carried out on the condition that the patient's vital signs and blood oxygenation are stable and he or she can actively cooperate. The goal is to use physical training to increase muscle strength, promote respiratory function, and improve limb movement when patients can tolerate exercise.

Bedside limb exercises are suitable for severe patients whose pneumonia are stabilized, but have reduced cardiopulmonary function and physical activity. The goal is to use physical training to increase muscle strength and limb movement, and improve cardiopulmonary function when patients are tolerant to exercise. Select exercises that activate the joints, step training, etc.

Walk Training Once the patient is able to stand and balance, and has completed bedside step training, he or she can begin walk training with support 2–3 times per day, 5–10 min per session.

Balance training, including standing on one leg, cross-walking, horizontal walking, and others, can be alternated with walking training.

4.9.6.9 Resistance Exercise

Resistance training is suitable for mild cases or severe cases in remission with stabilized pneumonia but with an obvious decline in muscle strength. Low-intensity resistance training can be used during hospitalization, and self antigravity training such as sitting and standing, wall squats, wall pushes, or resistance training with elastic bands. Repeat each exercise 10–15 times for 2–3 sets, as long as the patient does not have dyspnea, pain, or severe fatigue. Blood oxygen needs to be monitored the entire time, and exercises requiring straining while holding the breath should be avoided.

4.10 Clinical Pharmacy Services for Hospitalized Patients

Yu Zhang, Yuyong Su and Xuefeng Cai

Pharmaceutical intervention is a key component of COVID-19 treatment. Most severe and critical COVID-19 patients have underlying comorbidities and complicated medication regimens. Therefore, integrated pharmaceutical services are very important to ensure the safety of patients' medication in a comprehensive and timely manner during the epidemic.

4.10.1 Ensuring the Supply of Medications During the Epidemic

When responding to COVID-19 public health emergencies, ensuring the supply of medications is of great importance to improve medical treatment capabilities and support epidemic prevention and control. Drug supply is mainly ensured by drawing up a drug catalog based on diagnosis and treatment scheme and guidelines relevant to COVID-19, to maintain a timely, effective, and sufficient supply to meet the needs of clinical diagnosis and treatment.

4.10.2 Clinical Pharmacy Services for COVID-19 Diagnosis and Treatment

During the epidemic, clinical pharmacists rely on information technology to offer clinical pharmacy services, including prescription confirmation, medication consultations, pharmacy ward rounding, pharmacy consultation, and pharmaceutical care.

4.10.2.1 Examination and Verification of Prescription

Clinical pharmacists formulate prescription review standards for pharmaceuticals usage in COVID-19's diagnosis and treatment based on the drug instructions, COVID-19 related diagnosis and treatment scheme, evidence-based medical data, and so forth. The clinical pharmacists keep the rules for updated review in a software database for reasonable usage of the medications, warn clinicians about reasonable use of medications when medical orders are issued, and promptly intercept medical orders which call for unreasonable use of medication. Clinical pharmacists review medical orders that have already been issued mainly for drug interactions, duplicate medications, and use in special populations. During the epidemic, an online system for communicating about unreasonable medical orders should be established to ensure that communication between doctors and pharmacists is timely and efficient. Clinical pharmacists keep records of unreasonable medical orders upon review, and give feedback to clinicians by summarizing frequent problems.

4.10.2.2 Medication Consultation

4.10.2.2.1 Clinical Drug Usage Consultations

Antiviral drugs used during the epidemic are not standard stock medicines in hospitals, and some clinicians lack experience with using them. Clinical pharmacists can provide consultation for clinicians in terms of usage, dosage, indication, mechanism, and usage in special groups. Nurse inquiries mainly entail a drug's administration, compatibility, infusion rate, infusion stability, and storage. In order to reduce contact between personnel, inquiries can be made via Internet, phone, or video. Clinical pharmacists should summarize high-frequency inquiries, and write up the usage information for clinical reference.

4.10.2.2.2 Medication Consultation for Patients

Most hospitalized COVID-19 patients suffer from underlying diseases, and their drug regimens are specialized. Providing patients with specific medication consultations can ensure medication usage safe and effective. Inquiries may include medication usage, precautions, adverse reactions, and food–drug interactions. Clinical pharmacists should respect patients, protect patients' privacy, help patients articulate their inquiries patiently and meticulously and use plain language to answer patients' questions correctly during the medication consultation. The hospital's online consultation program can be used to provide patients with medication consultation, as well as WeChat, telephone, or other means.

4.10.2.3 Pharmacy Ward Rounds

Clinical pharmacists should participate in pharmacy ward rounding with protective gear. Pharmacy ward rounds include pharmaceutical consultation, evaluation of patients' compliance with a drug regimen, evaluation of medication efficacy, patient drug education, and monitoring of adverse reactions. Clinical pharmacists evaluate treatment efficacy based on the patient's examination indicators and posttreatment symptoms and signs if with improvement then formulate a monitoring plan, provide doctors with timely advice on the adjustment of the drug treatment plan. Communicate with nurses, about administration methods (such as drip rate). Drug storage (such as keep away from light), the order of drug administrating, and so on. Records are kept for clinical references.

4.10.2.4 Pharmacological Diagnostic Consultation and MDT Discussion

About 10% of COVID-19 patients have secondary infections during hospitalization, and most patients receive empirical antibacterial therapy [31]. Clinical pharmacist participation in anti-infective pharmaceutical diagnostic consultations can promote the rational use of antibacterial drugs and enhance the effectiveness of anti-infective treatments. During consultations regarding anti-infective pharmaceuticals, clinical pharmacists must determine whether there is a bacterial infection, find the source of the secondary infection, and recommend suitable antibacterial drugs based on the infection site, common pathogens, patient status, medication history, high-risk factors for drug resistance, etc., to formulate a dosing regimen based on antimicrobial PK/PD modeling. Clinical pharmacists and clinicians form an MDT team to improve drug treatment plans for difficult and critical COVID-19 cases.

4.10.2.5 Pharmaceutical Care

Pharmaceutical care of COVID-19 patients includes observation of medication efficacy, safety monitoring, evaluation of drug interactions, and adjustment of drug regimen for special populations. The major special populations are children, pregnant women, the elderly, mechanically ventilated patients, patients with liver and kidney dysfunction, patients undergoing extracorporeal membrane oxygenation or renal replacement therapy, and other patients whose physiological characteristics and pharmaceutical combinations will alter a drug's pharmacokinetics and affect the efficacy. Therefore, clinical pharmacists must make recommendations to personalize treatment based on the patients' special physiological characteristics and medication risks.

Inhibition of viral replication is the key to control the development of COVID-19. Drugs for this purpose are the most frequently utilized in treatment. See Attachment 1 for the main points of pharmaceutical care of drugs in this class [32–38]. In the present, there is no drug confirmed to be effective against COVID-19. As progress is made in COVID-19 research, clinical trials of drugs for COVID-19 are also continuously adjusted. The latest version of the diagnosis and treatment plan developed by the National Health Commission of the People's Republic of China [39] mainly recommends the use of α-interferon, Lopinavir/Ritonavir, Ribavirin, Chloroquine Phosphate, and Arbidol. The plan also states that the use of three or more antiviral drugs concurrently is not recommended.

4.10.3 Adverse Reaction Monitoring

In the treatment of COVID-19, attention should be paid to adverse drug reactions, especially those of clinical trial and clinical research medication. Pharmacists should pay attention to identify symptoms of the disease, and use proper judgment on the causes and effects of adverse drug reactions. According to the circumstances, pharmacists should report adverse reactions, actively monitor pharmaceutical applications, issue early clinical warnings, pay attention to the prognosis of adverse reactions, analyze drug safety information, offer clinical feedback, and ensure the safety of clinical drug regimens.

Attachment 1. Essentials of Antiviral Drug Use and Monitoring

1. **α-Interferon (Nebulization)**
   (a) Possible mechanism of action: By inhibiting the synthesis of viral RNA and protein, cells are induced to produce antiviral proteins, thereby exerting antiviral effects.
   (b) Metabolic pathway: Catabolism in the lungs.
   (c) ADR: Aerosol inhalation has fewer adverse reactions, though low fever is seen occasionally.
   (d) Precautions: Ultrasonic nebulization is not recommended, but jet nebulizers may be considered. Care should be taken to avoid contact with eyes during nebulization. Nebulization in a negative pressure ward is recommended in order to avoid aerosol induction.
   (e) Drug interactions: Reduction in the clearance rate of theophylline can result in theophylline poisoning. It is necessary to monitor the blood concentration of theophylline and adjust the dose. Combination with antiepileptic drugs, antituberculosis drugs, and other drugs that have an impact on liver function poses a potential risk of liver poisoning. Take care to check liver function in people with a history of liver disease. Combination with Zidovudine can increase the incidence of adverse reactions.
   (f) Contraindications for combined use: Do not nebulize simultaneously with chymotrypsin, acetylcysteine, or ipratropium bromide.
   (g) Adjustment of drug regimen: Use of ultrasonic nebulization should be avoided in patients on mechanical ventilation. It is not necessary to adjust drug dosage while patients are receiving ECMO and RRT.
   (h) Contraindications: Known allergies to interferon products; history of angina pectoris, myocardial infarction, or other serious cardiovascular diseases; serious conditions those do not tolerate this drug's side effects; epilepsy and other central nervous system dysfunction.
2. **Lopinavir/Ritonavir**
   (a) Possible mechanism of action: Inhibition of the 3CLpro's protease activity of SARS-Cov.
   (b) Metabolic pathways and metabolic enzymes: Liver CYP3A enzyme metabolism.
   (c) ADR: Diarrhea, nausea and vomiting, hypertriglyceridemia, impaired liver function, etc.
   (d) Precautions: The tablets can be taken before or after meals. The tablets should be swallowed in total, not be chewed, broken, or crushed. The oral solution contains ethanol and propylene glycol and should be taken together with food. Oral liquid can be used for tube-fed patients with PVC and silicone tubes. Polyurethane tubes cannot be used for the tube-fed patients.
   (e) Drug interactions: Lopinavir/Ritonavir co-administered with drugs metabolized via CYP3A (such as dihydropyridine, calcium channel blockers, HMG-CoA reductase inhibitors, immunosuppressants, and PDE5 inhibi-

tors) can lead to increased plasma concentrations of these drugs. Combination of Lopinavir/Ritonavir with voriconazole may reduce the blood drug concentrations of voriconazole.

(f) Contraindication for combinational usage: It is contraindicated to be used together with medications such as Amiodarone, Fusidic Acid, Colchicine, Cisapride, Quetiapine, Lovastatin, Simvastatin, Midazolam, Triazolam, and Ergot Alkaloids.

(g) Adjustment of drug regimen: Oral liquid can be selected for patients on mechanical ventilation. The dosage should be increased when using ECMO. There is no need to adjust the dosage while on RRT.

(h) Contraindications: Allergy to Lopinavir, Ritonavir, or any excipients; severe liver dysfunction.

3. **Favipiravir**
   (a) Possible mechanism of action: Selective inhibition of RNA polymerase associated with viral replication.
   (b) Metabolic pathway: Metabolized by the liver.
   (c) ADR: Increased blood uric acid, diarrhea, decreased neutrophil count, increased AST and ALT, etc.
   (d) Precautions: Reproductive toxicity. Can pass through the placenta and breast milk. Lactating women should discontinue breastfeeding.
   (e) Drug interactions: Theophylline can increase the bioavailability of Favipiravir. Favipiravir can increase the bioavailability of acetaminophen by 1.79 times, with elevated uric acid level in the blood when combinated with pyrazinamide, and increased blood concentration of repaglinide that can induce risk of hypoglycemia.
   (f) Adjustment of drug regimen: Not necessary in mechanically ventilated patients.
   (g) Contraindications: Pregnancy or possible pregnancy; allergic to favipiravir
4. **Ribavirin**
   (a) Possible mechanism of action: Inhibition of viral RNA polymerase and mRNA guanosine transferase.
   (b) Metabolic pathway: Intrahepatic metabolism.
   (c) ADR: Can cause hemolytic anemia and heart damage. There are also reports of low electrolyte disturbances and central nervous system toxicity.
   (d) Precautions: Ribavirin has reproductive toxicity, can pass through the placenta and breast milk. Men and women taking this product should use contraception prior to starting, while taking, and at least 6 months after discontinuing the medication. Lactating women should discontinue breastfeeding.
   (e) Drug interactions: Combination with Zidovudine can lead to increased drug toxicity. Combination with nucleoside reverse transcriptase inhibitors can lead to increased risk of adverse reactions related to mitochondrial poisoning (lactic acidosis, pancreatitis, and liver failure).

(f) Adjustment of drug regimen: Not necessary for patients on mechanical ventilation and those using ECMO. Hemodialysis patients should be administered 1/2 the original dose. No adjustment required in CRRT patients.
(g) Contraindications: Pregnancy, autoimmune hepatitis, allergy to ribavirin.

5. **Chloroquine Phosphate**
   (a) Possible mechanism of action: Inhibition of coronavirus binding to ACE2 receptors in human cells; inhibition of interferon and interleukin-6 production and release.
   (b) Metabolic pathway: Liver metabolism.
   (c) ADR: Arrhythmia, adverse gastrointestinal reactions, blood cell decline, rash, and impaired vision. The most serious ADR is cardiotoxicity, which can cause cardiac arrest. Long-term or large doses can cause irreversible retinopathy.
   (d) Precautions: Electrocardiogram must be normal before starting the treatment. Pay close attention to adverse reactions after administration. Discontinue immediately in case of intolerable toxic side effects. Pay attention to changes in the patient's vision during treatment. Observe the patient's mental state for psychological abnormalities, depression, etc.
   (e) Drug interactions: Monitor liver function closely when combined with Lopinavir/Ritonavir, Ribavirin, Arbidol, Favipiravir, as these drugs all exhibit hepatotoxicity. Closely monitor adverse cardiac reactions when used with Arbidol.
   (f) Contraindications for combined use: Moxifloxacin, azithromycin, and other drugs may cause prolonged Q–T interval.
   (g) Adjustment of drug regimen: Not required in patients on mechanical ventilation. RRT patients can be partially cleared by hemodialysis.
   (h) Contraindications: Pregnancy; known allergy to 4-aminoquinine compounds; arrhythmia (such as conduction block), chronic heart disease; end-stage chronic liver and kidney disease; known retinal disease, diminished hearing, or hearing loss; known mental disorder; skin disease (rash, dermatitis, psoriasis); glucose-6-phosphate dehydrogenase deficiency.
6. **Arbidol**
   (a) Possible mechanism of action: Inhibition of fusion of viral lipid membranes with human cells; induction of interferon production in human cells, which in turn induces production of multiple antiviral proteins.
   (b) Metabolic pathways and metabolic enzymes: Through liver CYP3A4 enzyme metabolism.
   (c) ADR: Mainly nausea, diarrhea, dizziness, and elevated serum transaminase.
   (d) Precautions: Safety in patients over 65 years of age has not been established.
   (e) Drug interactions: Possible interactions between CYP3A4 and UGT1A9 substrates, inhibitors, and inducers. Monitor carefully if used with Propofol and Zidovudine. Liver enzymes and jaundice may increase when used with Lopinavir.
   (f) Adjustment of drug regimen: Not necessary in mechanically ventilated patients.
   (g) Contraindications: Allergic to arbidol.

4.11 Psychological Intervention to Patients

Jian Luo

4.11.1 Psychological Reaction and Psychiatric Symptoms of COVID-19 Patients

After diagnosis with COVID-19, patients often feel annoyed, self-blame, anxiety, fear, have insomnia, nightmares, sadness and despration, sensitivity, paranoia, irritability and quickness to anger, and may become aggressive [40]. Suspected patients often face unknown fear and helplessness while isolating and waiting for test results [41]. Psychological evaluation in the isolation ward shows that about 48% of COVID-19 patients have psychological reactions at the beginning of admission, most of which are emotional reactions under stress [42]. Deliration occurs in a high proportion of critical patients. One case of encephalitis caused by COVID-19 infection was reported, accompanied by symptoms such as unconsciousness and irritability.

4.11.2 Establishing Dynamic Psychological Assessment and Early Warning

All patients undergo dynamic psychological assessments weekly after admission and before discharge. Mental health self-assessment tools: Mental health self-assessment (SRQ-20), depression screening (PHQ-9), generalized anxiety screening (GAD-7). Mental health scale: Hamilton Depression Scale (HAM-D), Hamilton Anxiety Scale (HAMA), Positive and Negative Syndrome Scale (PANSS) in the special environment of the isolation ward, patients are advised to complete the self-assessment questionnaire on a mobile phone under guidance. You can also conduct interviews and assessments in person or via voice connection. For patients who have breathing difficulties or difficulty completing the self-assessment questionnaire on a mobile phone, we recommended using the four-question method of the PHQ-9 (If there are two or more positive answers, further psychological assessment is required). For in-person screening, use the GAD-7 four-question method (if the answers are all positive, further psychological assessment is required). The patient can answer by simply nodding or shaking their head [43].

4.11.3 Counseling Intervention

4.11.3.1 Intervention Principles

For patients with positive psychological assessment results, non-pharmacological psychological interventions are recommended. Relaxation breathing, mindfulness, meditation, music therapy, and so on can be used for psychological self-regulation [44]. If conditions permit, psychological counselors can offer individualized one-on-one counseling. Commonly used psychological counseling methods include progressive whole-body muscle relaxation, cognitive transformation therapy, experiential transformation, and existential purpose therapies. For patients in whom non-pharmacological intervention is not efficacious, use of drugs in combination with psychological intervention is recommended [42]. New antidepressants and anxiolytics, as well as benzodiazepines can be given to improve mood and sleep problems [40]. Second-generation antipsychotic drugs such as Olanzapine and Quetiapine improve hallucinations, delusions, and other psychotic symptoms [40].

4.11.3.2 Precautions When Using Psychotropic Drugs [40]

COVID-19 has a high incidence in middle-aged and elderly populations, and is often accompanied by underlying physical diseases such as hypertension and diabetes. Therefore, when selecting psychotropic drugs, drug interactions, and effects on respiration must be fully considered. Citalopram and Escitalopram are recommended for depression and anxiety, benzodiazepines such as Estazolam and Alprazolam for anxiety and sleep quality, and Olanzapine and Quetiapine for psychotic symptoms. Use psychotropic drugs with caution for patients who have dyspnea or respiratory failure.

4.12 Discharge Criteria and Patient Follow-Up

Ying Su

4.12.1 Discharge Criteria

According to the COVID-19 Diagnosis and Treatment Plan (Trial Version 7) issued by the National Health Commission of the People's Republic of China, the discharge criteria for COVID-19 patients are as follows:

1. Body temperature has returned to normal for more than 3 days.
2. Respiratory symptoms have improved significantly.
3. Lung imaging shows a significant improvement in acute exudative lesions.
4. Two consecutive sputum, nasopharyngeal swabs, or other respiratory tract specimens test negative for nucleic acid testing (sampling time at least 24 h apart).

Those who meet the above conditions can be discharged.

4.12.2 Medical Advice and Precautions for Hospital Discharge [45]

14-Day isolation and health monitoring are required for all patients discharged from the hospital.

It is recommended that patients return to the nearest hospital on the second and fourth weeks after discharge. The treatment hospital conducts a telephone follow-up interview one week after the patient is discharged to keep updating about the patient's physical and mental healthy status and make sure to remind the patient back to the hospital for follow-up examinations.

4.12.3 Home Isolation Precautions [46]

In general, all recovered and discharged patients should be transferred to a rehabilitation station in the jurisdiction of their home address for 2 weeks of isolation and observation. In special circumstances, such as older age, inability to take care of oneself, mental disorder, pregnancy, or other conditions not suitable for independent living in a rehabilitation station, home isolation can be applied for. The following precautions should be taken during home isolation:

1. Enhance health awareness, exercise properly, and ensure sufficient and early sleep to improve immunity.
2. If conditions permit, stay in a well-ventilated single room, and reduce close contact with family members.
3. Eat meals by dishes separately, maintain hand hygiene, and avoid outside activities.
4. Maintain good personal hygiene. Cover your mouth and nose with a tissue, your sleeve, or your elbow when coughing or sneezing. Wash your hands thoroughly, and do not touch your eyes, nose, or mouth with dirty hands.
5. If possible, avoid close contact with people who have symptoms of respiratory diseases (such as fever, cough, and sneezing).
6. Avoid crowded and confined spaces as much as possible. If unable to do so, wear a mask.
7. Avoid contact with wild animals, poultry, and livestock.
8. Adhere to safe eating habits. Meat and eggs should be fully cooked.
9. Pay close attention to symptoms such as fever and cough, and check your body temperature twice a day (morning and evening). If you have these symptoms, seek medical treatment immediately.

4.12.4 Follow-Up

The hospital arranges the physician for a telephone follow-up for the first week after discharge. The patient is instructed to go to the nearest hospital for an outpatient follow-up 2 and 4 weeks after discharge. Liver and kidney function tests and a blood routine test are recommended during the follow-up examination, as well as sputum or nasopharyngeal swab for viral nucleic acid testing, lung function assessment, and lung CT. At the third and sixth month after discharge, follow-up is conducted on the hospital's official WeChat platform.

Content of the first follow-up telephone interview is as follows:

4.12.4.1 Assessment of Clinical Symptomology

After discharge, ask if the patient has fever, cough, expectoration, dyspnea, shortness of breath after activity, fatigue, diarrhea, muscle aches, decreased muscle strength, etc.

4.12.4.2 Mental Health Assessment

Assessment based on the self-rating depression scale (SDS), self-rating anxiety scale (SAS), and Pittsburgh sleep questionnaire, etc.

4.12.5 Handling of Repeat Positive Patients

For the patients meeting discharge criteria, but positive with nucleic acid test again on follow-up which might be related to the retention of initial specimens and the detection of false negatives, we recommend:

1. Isolate according to the standards for patients diagnosed with COVID-19.
2. Decide whether to continue initially effective antiretroviral therapy according to clinical symptoms and lung CT findings.
3. Discharge after lung imaging further improved, and the sputum and nasopharyngeal swab are nucleic acid negative for three times (24 h apart).
4. Observe discharged patients according to the above isolation method and follow-up requirements.

References

1. Notice on Printing and Distribution of COVID-19 Diagnosis and Treatment Plan (Trial Version 7) issued by the General Office of National Health Commission of the People's Republic of China and the Office of State Administration of Traditional Chinese Medicine on March 3, 2020.
2. Notice on Printing and Distribution of Diagnosis and Treatment Plans for Severe and Critical COVID-19 Cases (Trial Version 2) issued by the General Office of National Health Commission of the People's Republic of China and the Office of State Administration of Traditional Chinese Medicine on February 14, 2020.
3. Regulations on Strengthening the Management of Fever Clinics at Present Stage issued by the medical treatment team of Wuhan Municipal Headquarters for COVID-19 Prevention and Control on March 13, 2020.
4. Notice on Expediting the Elimination of Suspected COVID-19 Cases in Wuhan issued by the treatment team of Wuhan Municipal Headquarters for COVID-19 Prevention and Control on February 21, 2020.
5. Urgent Notice on Implementing Best Practices for Admission and Observation of Patients at Fever Clinics issued by the medical treatment team of Wuhan Municipal Headquarters for COVID-19 Prevention and Control on February 18, 2020.
6. Notice on Implementing the Plan for Strengthening Triage Management of Patients at Fever Clinics in Wuhan issued by the medical treatment team of Wuhan Municipal Headquarters for COVID-19 Prevention and Control on February 7, 2020.

7. Zhou F, Yu T, Du R, et al. Clinical course and risk factors for mortality of adult inpatients with COVID-19 in Wuhan, China: a retrospective cohort study. The Lancet. 2020; https://doi.org/10.1016/S0140-6736(20)30566-3.
8. Wang D, Hu B, Hu C, Zhu F, Liu X, Zhang J, et al. Clinical characteristics of 138 hospitalized patients with 2019 novel coronavirus–infected pneumonia in Wuhan. China. JAMA. 2020;323(11):1061–9.
9. Wu Z, McGoogan JM. Characteristics of and important lessons from the coronavirus disease 2019 (COVID-19) outbreak in China: summary of a report of 72 314 cases from the Chinese Center for Disease Control and Prevention. JAMA. 2020; https://doi.org/10.1001/jama.2020.2648.
10. Chen N, Zhou M, Dong X, Qu J, Gong F, Han Y, et al. Epidemiological and clinical characteristics of 99 cases of 2019 novel coronavirus pneumonia in Wuhan, China: a descriptive study. The Lancet. 2020;395(10223):507–13.
11. Huang C, Wang Y, Li X, Ren L, Zhao J, Hu Y, et al. Clinical features of patients infected with 2019 novel coronavirus in Wuhan, China. The Lancet. 2020;395(10223):497–506.
12. Poston JT, Patel BK, Davis AM. Management of critically ill adults with COVID-19. JAMA. https://doi.org/10.1001/jama.2020.4914.
13. Luo Y, Zhong M. Standardized diagnosis and treatment of colorectal cancer during the outbreak of corona virus disease 2019 in Renji hospital. Zhonghua Wei Chang Wai Ke Za Zhi. 2020;23(03):211–6.
14. Francois L, Angus Derek C. Toward universal deployable guidelines for the care of patients with COVID-19. JAMA. https://doi.org/10.1001/jama.2020.5110.
15. Surviving Sepsis Campaign. COVID-19 Guidelines. Published March 20, 2020. https://www.sccm.org/SurvivingSepsisCampaign/Guidelines/COVID-19.
16. Military Medical Expert Group on the Front-line. Diagnosis and treatment protocol for novel Coronavirus disease from Military Medical Team supporting Wuhan (Trial Version 2). Chin J Tuberc Respir Dis. 2020;43:414–20.
17. Day M. Covid-19: ibuprofen should not be used for managing symptoms, say doctors and scientists. BMJ. 2020;368:m1086.
18. Feng B, Chen ZX, Jin LW, et al. Concerns about the Pharmacotherapeutics of COVID-19 based on the Essence of "Sputum Emboli". Pharmacy Today. 2020.
19. Liu Y, et al. The military supports the Hubei Medical Team's COVID-19 diagnosis and treatment plan (Provisional 1st Version). Chin J Tuberc Respir Dis. 2020;43:E024.
20. Zhang W, et al. Shanghai 2019; expert consensus on comprehensive treatment of COVID-19. Chin J Infect Dis. 2020;38:E016. https://doi.org/10.3760/cma.j.issn.1000-6680.2020.0016.
21. National Health Commission of the People's Republic of China, State Administration of Traditional Chinese Medicine. COVID-19 Diagnosis and Treatment Plan (Trial Version 7) [Z]. February 2020. GWBYH [2020] No. 184. http://www.nhc.gov.cn/yzygj/s7653p/202003/46c9294a7dfe4cef80dc7f5912eb1989.shtml.
22. Denga L, Li C, Zeng Q, et al. Arbidol combined with LPV/r versus LPV/r alone against Corona Virus Disease 2019: a retrospective cohort study. J Infect. 2020;12:51. https://doi.org/10.1016/j.jinf.2020.03.002.
23. Shanghai COVID-19 Clinical Treatment Expert Team. Shanghai 2019 expert consensus on comprehensive treatment of COVID-19. Chin J Infect Dis. 2020;38 https://doi.org/10.3760/cma.j.issn.1000-6680.2020.0016.. online pre-publication
24. Andre C. Kalil, Treating COVID-19—off-label drug use, compassionate use, and randomized clinical trials during pandemics. JAMA. Published online March 24, 2020. https://jamanetwork.com/. Accessed 27 Mar 2020.
25. Guarner F, Sanders ME, Eliakim R, et al. World gastroenterology organisation global guidelines: probiotics and prebiotics. J Clin Gastroenterol. 2017;51(2):468–81.
26. Wilkins T, Sequoia J. Probiotics for gastrointestinal conditions: a summary of the evidence. Am Fam Physician. 2017;96(3):170–8.
27. Toscano M, De Grandi R, Pastorelli L, Vecchi M, Drago L. A consumer's guide for probiotics: 10 goldees for a correct use. Dig Liver Dis. 2017;49(11):1177–84.

28. Reintam Blaser A, Starkopf J, Alhazzani W, et al. Early enteral nutrition in critically ill patients: ESICM clinical practice guidelines. Intensive Care Med. 2017;43(3):380–98.
29. McClave SA, DiBaise JK, Mullin GE, Martindale RG. ACG clinical guideline: nutrition therapy in the adult hospitalized patient. Am J Gastroenterol. 2016;111(3):315–35.
30. Singer P, Blaser AR, Berger MM, et al. ESPEN guideline on clinical nutrition in the intensive care unit. Clin Nutr. 2019;38(1):48–79.
31. Huang C, Wang Y, Li X, et al. Clinical features of patients infected with 2019 novel coronavirus in Wuhan, China. Lancet. 2020;395(10223):497–506.
32. Bian Y, Wang Y, Yang Y, et al. Rational use and pharmaceutical care of two antiviral drugs. Herald Med. 1–16. http://kns.cnki.net/kcms/detail/42.1293.R.20200203.1003.002.html.
33. Wang R, Xu Q, Lu L, et al. Pharmacological care strategy for antivirals in patients with COVID-19 complicated by underlying disorders. Chin J Hosp Pharmacy. 2020:1–9.
34. Matoulkova P, Pavek P, Maly J, et al. Cytochrome P450 enzyme regulation by glucocorticoids and consequences in terms of drug interaction. Expert Opin Drug Metab Toxicol. 2014;10(3):425–35.
35. Abdul-Aziz MH, Roberts JA. Antibiotic dosing during extracorporeal membrane oxygenation: does the system matter? Curr Opin Anaesthesiol. 2020;33(1):71–82.
36. Zhejiang Province Pharmaceutical Association. Guidance and recommendations for pharmaceutical monitoring in severe and critical COVID-19 patients (Trial) [EB/OL]. [2020-03-02].
37. Hubei Province Clinical Pharmaceutical Quality Control Center. Hubei Province guidelines for clinical pharmaceutical use in COVID-19 cases (Version 1) [EB/OL]. [2020-03-12].
38. Li L, Chen N, Kong L, et al. Antiviral therapeutics for 2019 novel coronavirus infection in special populations. Chin J Mod Appl Pharmacy. 2020;37(03):257–63.
39. National Health Commission of the People's Republic of China. COVID-19 diagnosis and treatment plan (Trial Version 7) GWBYH [2020] No. 184 [EB/OL]. [2020-03-03].
40. Psychiatry Branch of Chinese Medical Association, Psychiatrist branch of Chinese Medical Association. Recommendations for the use of psychotropic drugs in patients with new coronavirus pneumonia. Chin J Psychiatry. 2020;53(02):84–8. https://doi.org/10.3760/cma.j.cn113661-20200221-00045.
41. National Health Commission of the People's Republic of China. Guideline for psychological crisis intervention during 2019-nCoV. 26 Jan 2020. http://www.nhc.gov.cn/jkj/s3577/202001/6adc08b966594253b2b791be5c3b9467.shtml.
42. Mingliang J, Xu Q, Bin L, et al. Psychotropic drug intervention in patients with acute stress disorder caused by coronavirus disease 2019: a report of 2 cases. Chin J Nerv Mental Dis. 1–5. http://kns.cnki.net/kcms/detail/44.1213.R.20200228.0925.004.html.
43. Xu K, Cai H, Shen Y, et al. Management of corona virus disease-19 (COVID-19): the Zhejiang experience. J Zhejiang Univ (Med Sci). 1–12. http://kns.cnki.net/kcms/detail/33.1248.R.20200222.1417.002.html.
44. Fu X, Zhang X, Zhao Z. Psychological adjustment during outbreak of COVID-19 based on traditional Chinese medicine emotion therapy. Chin J Exp Tradit Med Formul. 1–6. https://doi.org/10.13422/j.cnki.syfjx.20201322.
45. Health management plan for discharged COVID-19 patients (Trial). http://www.gov.cn/zhengce/zhengceku/2020-03/15/content_5491535.htm.
46. Guidance on medical observation and control of infection for home isolation in the prevention and control of COVID-19 (Trial). http://www.nhc.gov.cn/yzygj/s7659/202002/cf80b05048584f8da9b4a54871c44b26.shtm.

Treatment of Critical COVID-19 Patients

5

Xiaomeng Zhang, Zhaohui Fu, and Weimin Xiao

Contents

The corresponding author of Sects. 5.1 and 5.2 is Zhaohui Fu, Email: 1334485308@qq.com
The corresponding author of Sect. 5.3 is Weimin Xiao, Email: xiaoweimin199968@163.com
The corresponding author of Sect. 5.4 is Xiaomeng Zhang, Email: 1161576293@qq.com
The corresponding author of Sect. 5.5 is Zhaohui Fu, Email: 1334485308@qq.com

X. Zhang
Department of Otolaryngology, Union Hospital, Tongji Medical College, Huazhong University of Science and Technology, Wuhan, China

Z. Fu (✉)
Critical Care Medicine, Union Hospital, Tongji Medical College, Huazhong University of Science and Technology, Wuhan, China

W. Xiao
Department of Anesthesiology, Union Hospital, Tongji Medical College, Huazhong University of Science and Technology, Wuhan, China

F. Cheng, Y. Zhang (eds.), *The Clinical Diagnosis and Treatment for New Coronavirus Pneumonia*, https://doi.org/10.1007/978-981-15-5975-4_5

5.1 Treatment Principles for the Critical COVID-19 Patients Admitted to ICU

Zhaohui Fu

Early identification of critical COVID-19 patients who meet one of the following conditions:

1. Suffering from respiratory failure that requires mechanical ventilation.
2. Suffering from shock.
3. Suffering from a combination of other organ dysfunctions requiring ICU monitoring and management.

5.1.1 Treatment of Critical Patients

5.1.1.1 Treatment Principles

On the basis of symptomatic treatment, active life support shall be applied to prevent organ dysfunctions. Treat underlying diseases, and actively prevent and treat complications.

5.1.1.2 Respiratory Support

For patients who fail to respond to common oxygen therapy, oxygenation with high-flow nasal cannula or noninvasive ventilator-based ventilation may be considered. Changes in the patient's respiratory status should be closely observed and tracheal intubation and invasive ventilation should be considered if the patient does not experience significant improvement within 1–2 h. Since some critical patients with severe hypoxia may not have significant symptoms of respiratory distress, careful assessment is required. The dynamic changes in HR, RR, BP, SPO2, blood gas analysis, etc. should be closely monitored, and attention may be paid to whether patients are using accessory respiratory muscles for breathing. If the patient's condition does not improve, or with altered mental status, hemodynamic instability, failure to remove airway secretions, intolerance to noninvasive ventilation, etc., tracheal intubation and invasive ventilation should be considered as early as possible.

A "lung-protective strategy" for invasive mechanical ventilation, i.e., the administration of a lower tidal volume (predicted body weight 4–8 mL/kg) and a lower inspiratory pressure (plateau pressure <30 cm H_2O), should be applied to reduce ventilator-associated lung injury. High PEEP can be applied appropriately in case of ensuring a plateau pressure $\leq$35 cm H_2O. Human–machine dyssynchrony may occur for many patients. Adequate sedation, analgesia, and muscle relaxant therapy may be considered. Closed suction tubing can be used, and fiber optic bronchoscopy will be performed in accordance with the patient's airway secretions.

For patients with severe ARDS, lung recruitment is recommended. Prone position ventilation should be performed for more than12 h/day. For patients with poor mechanical ventilation in the prone position, if conditions allowed, extracorporeal membrane oxygenation (ECMO) should be considered as soon as possible. ECMO indications: (1) In case of $FiO_2 > 90\%$, oxygenation index less than 80 mmHg, with a duration of more than 3–4 h; (2) airway plateau pressure $\geq$35 cm H_2O. For patients with only respiratory failure, VV-ECMO mode will be preferred; if circulatory support is required, VA-ECMO mode shall be selected when the underlying disease has been controlled, cardiopulmonary function shows signs of recovery, and withdrawal tests can be initiated.

5.1.1.3 Circulatory Support

On the basis of adequate fluid resuscitation, microcirculation shall be improved, vasoactive drugs shall be used, and changes in patient's blood pressure, heart rate, and urine volume as well as lactate and base excess in their arterial blood gas analysis shall be closely monitored. Noninvasive or invasive hemodynamic monitoring shall be performed, such as ultrasonic Doppler, echocardiography, invasive blood pressure, or PiCCO monitoring, when necessary. Identify the type of shock in patients to guide fluid replacement therapy.

5.1.1.4 Renal Failure and Renal Replacement Therapy

The cause of renal impairment in critical patients should be figured out actively. In the treatment of patients with renal failure, attention should be paid to fluid balance, acid–base balance, and electrolyte balance. For severe patients, CRRT can be considered for treatment. Indications include (1) hyperkalemia, (2) acidosis, (3) pulmonary edema or water overload, and (4) fluid management in case of multiple organ dysfunctions.

5.1.1.5 Nutritional Support

Patients admitted to the ICU should undergo nutritional risk screening using the Nutritional Risk Scale. ICU patients are most at risk of malnutrition, so nutritional support should be applied as early as possible. If the patient is able to eat, eating by mouth is preferred. If not, EN should be performed as early as possible (within 48 h). If EN cannot be administered, PN is recommended (3–7 days). For patients with enteral nutritional intolerance, Erythromycin and other gastrointestinal motility drugs can be considered. In case of the poor effects of gastrointestinal motility drugs, jejunal feeding can be considered. PN should be considered in the absence of any effective attempt to improve EN tolerance, and regimen should be individualized with all-in-one formula as preferred. In the process of enteral nutrition support, gastrointestinal function such as gastric residual volume should be monitored, and attention should be paid to whether the patient has gastrointestinal symptoms such as diarrhea, nausea, and vomiting, and changes in blood glucose and electrolytes should be monitored. Patients with long-term parenteral nutrition support should be monitored for changes in blood glucose, electrolytes, liver, and renal function.

5.1.1.6 Convalescent Plasma Therapy

It applies to patients with rapid disease progression, severe, and critical types of illness.

5.1.1.7 Blood-Purifying Therapy

The blood purification system includes plasma exchange, adsorption, perfusion, blood/plasma filtration, etc., which can remove inflammatory factors and block the "cytokine storm," thus mitigating the damage of inflammatory response to the body. It can be used for the early and mid-term treatment of cytokine storm in severe and critical patients.

5.1.1.8 Immunotherapy

For patients with extensive involvement and severe patients, and those with elevated IL-6 levels, tocilizumab treatment can be used. The first dose is 4–8 mg/kg (the recommended dose is 400 mg, diluted to 100 mL with 0.9% normal saline), infusion for more than 1 h; for patients with poor response to the first dose, an additional dose can be administered after 12 h (same dosage as the previous one). At the most maximum of 800 mg be aware of allergic reactions. It is contraindicated for patients with active infections such as tuberculosis.

5.1.1.9 Other Therapeutic Measures

For patients with progressive deterioration of oxygenation parameters, rapid imaging progression, and hyperactive body inflammation, glucocorticoids can be used in a short period of time (3–5 days) as appropriate, with the recommended dose not exceeding the equivalent of 1–2 mg/kg/day. It should be noted that larger doses of glucocorticoids will delay the clearance of coronavirus due to immunosuppressive effect; Xue Bi Jing (100 mL/time, twice daily) can be intravenously administered for treatment; intestinal microecological regulators can be used to maintain intestinal microecological balance and prevent secondary bacterial infection. Intravenous infusion of immunoglobulin can be considered for children with severe and critical symptoms as appropriate. Pregnant women with severe or critical COVID-19 should actively terminate their pregnancy, and cesarean section is preferred.

5.2 Anti-shock Therapy

Zhaohui Fu

For COVID-19 patients, shock is as one of the diagnostic criteria for critical illness, and also a sign of critical condition. With sudden increase of heart rate for more than 20% from baseline or the decrease of blood pressure greater than 20% from baseline, and accompanied by poor skin perfusion and decreased urine volume, the patient should be closely observed for septic shock, gastrointestinal bleeding, or heart failure. Meanwhile, we should quickly identify the type of shock in patients at an early stage.

The latest autopsy pathological changes in COVID-19 patients demonstrated visible degeneration and necrosis of myocardial cells in their heart, and infiltration of a few monocytes, lymphocytes, and/or neutrophils in the interstitium. Laboratory tests may reveal an increase in indicators such as TNI and CKMB, all of which suggest that the virus may cause myocardial damage. We found that some patients may be present with severe viral myocarditis or even cardiogenic shock during treatment. Patients with a combination of underlying diseases such as coronary heart disease, hypertension, and diabetes, may suffer from acute myocardial infarction. It resulted in more complex clinical pictures of such patients. Therefore, patients should undergo dynamic monitoring with ECG, myocardial enzyme spectrum, high-sensitivity troponin, B-type natriuretic peptide for identification, and, if necessary, coronary angiography can be performed to confirm the diagnosis. Bedside B-ultrasound, PICCO, etc. should be performed at an early stage for the assessment of changes in the patient's cardiac function. Patients with cardiogenic shocks, such as showing decreased CI, pulmonary congestion, and shock should be actively treated with anti-shock management. If the patient is induced by acute myocardial infarction, antiplatelet, and PCI treatment should be considered as early as possible. If the patient suffers from myocardial damage caused by COVID-19 viruses, drugs can be considered for nourishing the myocardium, among which dopamine, dobutamine, and other drugs can increase myocardial contractility, and in severe cases, treatments including IABP, VA-ECMO, etc. may also be considered.

Hypovolemic shock can be caused by inadequate fluid intake at the early stage, strict fluid restriction due to severe ARDS, and negative balance in COVID-19 patients. Autopsy pathological changes in COVID-19 patients have suggested different degrees of degeneration, necrosis, and shedding of the mucosal epithelium of the esophagus, stomach, and intestine, so gastrointestinal bleeding is also one of their common complications. Hypovolemic shock can also be frequently observed in patients with gastrointestinal bleeding. Dynamically monitoring the blood routine coagulation function, blood gas analysis, etc. should be performed. Monitoring CVP, PICCO with bedside B-ultrasound and other identification and monitoring and management of patient volume may be considered. Active fluid resuscitation, transfusion of blood products, etc. can be pursued to correct shock. If gastrointestinal bleeding is difficult to be controlled by medical treatment, digestive endoscopic hemostasis, or even surgical treatment can be considered.

COVID-19 patients are prone to sepsis and septic shock. According to the latest diagnostic criteria for sepsis 3.0, sepsis is defined as life-threatening organ dysfunction caused by a dysregulated host response against infection. The clinical diagnostic criterion for sepsis is based on SOFA score ≥2 with coinfection. Septic shock is a severe form of sepsis, and the clinical diagnostic criteria are that patients with sepsis have persistent hypotension after adequate fluid resuscitation and require vasopressors to maintain mean arterial pressure above 65 mmHg and blood lactate above 2 mmol/L. Septic shock can be quickly identified by the means of qSOFA score, etc. Treatment of septic shock should begin with adequate fluid resuscitation (fluid resuscitation with crystalloids is preferred), improvement of microcirculation, and usage of vasoactive agents (norepinephrine is preferred). Epinephrine is recommended when more vasoconstrictors are needed to maintain adequate blood pressure. Changes in patient's blood pressure, heart rate, and urine output, as well as lactate and base excess on arterial blood gas analysis should be closely monitored, and if necessary, noninvasive or invasive hemodynamic monitoring such as Doppler echocardiography, echocardiography, as well as invasive blood pressure or continuous cardiac output (PICCO) monitoring should be performed. During treatment, attention should be paid to fluid balance strategies to avoid overdose and underdose. Precautions for the treatment of septic shock: in the process of fluid resuscitation for patients with septic shock, lactate and lactate clearance rate can be used as indicators to determine the prognosis; crystalloids are the preferred resuscitation fluid for septic shock, and 30 mL/kg (body weight) of crystalloids should be rapidly infused within 1–2 h; hydroxyethyl starch is not recommended for fluid resuscitation; albumin can be considered for fluid resuscitation; the initial goal of vasoconstrictor drug therapy is for MAP close to 65 mmHg. Shock in patients at the early stage may be considered to be caused by viruses, and antiviral drugs can be considered and antibacterial drugs are selected based on PCT and WBC and etiology of the patients. Patients at the later stage are prone to bacterial or even fungal infections, and a comprehensive strategy may be considered. Sputum and blood microbiological tests should be performed as early as possible. If the effect of antibiotics is poor before drug sensitivity results have been obtained, the drug-resistant bacteria should be covered based on the situation of drug-resistant bacteria in our hospital.

COVID-19 patients showing shock symptoms are the signal for critical illness. The clinical picture of patients varies during treatment, so quick identification and active treatment are required. During the treatment, patients may experience ARDS aggravation, AKI, etc., and mechanical ventilation or even CRRT should be considered based on the condition. For patients with suboptimal shock correction, noninvasive or invasive hemodynamic monitoring such as Doppler echocardiography, echocardiography, as well as invasive blood pressure or continuous cardiac output (PiCCO) monitoring should be performed as early as possible. This will help us identify the type of shock at early stage to provide guidance on fluid resuscitation and treatment, which is important in managing the fluid balance of patients.

5.3 Tracheal Intubation

Weimin Xiao

5.3.1 Emergency Plan and Technical Process of Urgent Tracheal Intubation for COVID-19 Patients

Indications for urgent intubation for confirmed/clinically diagnosed/suspected cases in fever clinics and isolation ward areas:

1. It is manifested as severe hypoxemia without improvement or even deterioration of the condition under high-flow nasal cannula oxygen therapy or mechanical ventilation (the indications of BIPAP ventilator are patients with blood oxygen saturation less than 93%, no improvement of shortness of breath R > 30 beats/min, and conscious and cooperative patients under oxygen inhalation of 3–5 L/min).
2. Those who cannot clear respiratory secretions by themselves and need repeated suctioning due to significant amount of respiratory secretions.
3. Patients who are unable to wear a mask or nasal cannula due to facial trauma.
4. Patients with cardiorespiratory arrest.

5.3.2 Ward Preparations for Intubated Patients

Personnel preparation: Ask the doctor in charge and/or the medical personnel and nurses who are familiar with the usage and maintenance of ventilator as well as the operation of sputum suctioning for assistance.

Material Preparation:

1. Patients should fast for more than 6 h.
2. Sign the Informed Consent.
3. Open the venous access (with indwelling needles, 20G or above) and three-way valve, and connect to 0.9% normal saline.
4. Monitor vital signs (ECG, oxygen saturation, and blood pressure).
5. Connect the invasive ventilator with power supply, oxygen, screw pipe and membrane lung, and adjust the parameters of the respirator.
6. Reserve oxygen pillows full of oxygen for replacement.
7. Connect suction devices (negative pressure suction head, suction apparatus, connecting tube, and closed suction tube).
8. Prepare doctor's prescription in advance and prepare sedatives.

5.3.3 Precautions for Tracheal Intubation by Anesthesiologists

1. Reconfirm the indications of tracheal intubation, and know the patient's age, gender, weight, and complications upon notice via telephone.
2. Check the ventilator to set parameters properly, make sure the venous access is opened and evaluate the airway condition.
3. To reduce the risk of exposure, it is recommended that a trained and experienced anesthesiologist complete all the operations alone.
4. In order to reduce the cough caused by tracheal intubation and the spread of pathogens, moderate sedation, and intubation with adequate muscle relaxants are recommended.
5. For patients with unpredictable difficult airway and unsuccessful tracheal intubation for three times, laryngeal masks will be placed instead.

5.3.4 Protection Measures During Tracheal Intubation

Take Level-III medical protection measures:

Ensure good personal protection according to hospital requirements. For details, please see the manual "User Instructions for COVID-19 Protective Equipment".

Protocol for donning PPE: Disinfect both hands → put on a surgical cap → put on a medical protective mask → put on goggles/face shield/medical mask with eye shield → put on isolation gown/protective suit → put on shoe covers → put on gloves.

Protocol for removing PPE: Remove shoe covers → remove gloves → disinfect hands → remove isolation gown/protective suit → disinfect both hands → remove goggles/face shield → disinfect hands → remove medical protective mask → disinfect both hands → remove disposable round cap → disinfect hands/wash hands → replace medical protective mask and disposable working cap.

Avoid vibrating while removing PPE: After the protective suit is removed, roll it up from the inner surface and place it in the yellow garbage bin. The protective gear shall be discarded into the double-layer yellow garbage bags and placed in designated areas.

Those who go to the infected area or intubate for the suspected COVID-19 cases shall be properly disinfected before reentering the operating room. It is strictly prohibited to leave the contaminated area without removing personal protective equipment and take any used protective suit back to the operating room.

5.3.5 Pre-intubation Preparations

Antifogging: Antifogging is of paramount importance, otherwise rapid and accurate tracheal intubation will be impossible. It is recommended to perform antifogging before arriving at the fever clinics or isolation ward areas. Treat as follows:

1. Spray goggles with antifogging agent. Doctors wearing glasses should spray their glasses for antifogging at the same time.

2. Application of povidone-iodine: Pour the iodophor into the goggles, shake it from side to side, dump the excess iodophor after it lies flat, and let the goggles dry before use.
3. Apply hand sanitizer or detergent evenly to goggles with gauze and allow them to dry before use.

Narcotic drugs: Carry rapid onset general anesthesia-inducing drugs, such as Propofol, Etomidate, Fentanyl, and Rocuronium.

First aid drugs: Prepare ephedrine, atropine, epinephrine, salbutamol, aminophylline, etc.

Tracheal intubating appliances: Separately set up disposable visual laryngoscope lenses (discarded after use), primary tracheal tube bags, and appropriate models of tracheal tubes and laryngeal masks. After intubation, the visual laryngoscope stylet and video equipment will be disinfected in the contaminated area by UV light and then placed in a specific location of Intensive Care Unit (isolated storage).

5.3.6 Intubation Process

Before tracheal intubation, the patient monitoring equipment (ECG, blood pressure, and pulse oxygen saturation), intubation equipment (visual laryngoscope, oropharyngeal airway, tracheal tube, intubation stylet), and auxiliary respiratory equipment (respiratory balloon, mask) must be rechecked, various instrument circuits (at the head side of the patient), oxygen supply equipment and sputum suction equipment should be sorted out, and rescue drugs should be extracted for future use.

Preoxygenation before induction: Preoxygenation with 100% FiO_2 for 5 min through mask with oxygen storage bag, breathing mask, BIPAP ventilator, etc. [1]. High-flow preoxygenation can be administered through a mask when the patient is awake; oxygen flow can be increased in the case of BIPAP ventilator, and pressure-assisted ventilation should be avoided as much as possible before unconsciousness occurs to the patient. Patients with severe COVID-19, especially young children, obese, or pregnant patients, may see a rapid decrease in pulse oxygen saturation during intubation.

Anesthesia induction process (at least one nurse or doctor in the isolation ward area is needed to participate during the whole process):

1. Patients with unknown history at fever clinic will be treated under the condition of nonfasting.
2. For patients in the intensive care unit, airway assessment is not possible due to wearing the BIPAP ventilator on arrival to the ward. It is recommended to not remove their breathing masks for airway assessment and treat them under the condition of difficult airway. First, use Propofol 0.5–1 mg/kg [2], and observe the change in the patient's oxygen saturation under the condition of increased sedation (confrontations between insufficient sedation and noninvasive ventilator are common in the ward). When the saturation rises, use Propofol (60–80 mg)

again in combination of Rocuronium 0.9–1.2 mg/kg [2] and Fentanyl 2–4 μg/kg, while ensuring that BIPAP ventilator should not be withdrawn at this point.

Rapid intubation: Make sure the muscle relaxant works after 60–90 s of administration, and then quickly remove the respiratory mask of oxygen therapy or BIPAP ventilator and place the visual laryngoscope (preferred) [3] or common laryngoscope (disposable) to complete the intubation as fast as possible. It is recommended that the anesthesiologist perform the intubation alone, and, if necessary, some nurses can assist according to instructions from the anesthesiologist (nurses can help to deliver the catheter, pull out the stylet, and deliver pad, syringe, adhesive plaster, etc.), to ensure the successful completion of tracheal intubation.

Determination of depth of tracheal tube: The depth of tracheal tube for patients with severe pulmonary lesions cannot be determined through auscultatory breathing sound. It is recommended to observe the degree of thoracic fluctuation, respiratory waveform of ventilator, and respiratory parameters for comprehensive judgment. If conditions permit, end-tidal carbon dioxide or fiber optic microscopy can be used to determine the position of the tracheal tube [4], or use bedside ultrasonography to indirectly determine the position of the tracheal tube by checking whether it is mistakenly inserted into the esophagus. Auscultation is not recommended to determine the depth of tracheal tube, and bedside chest radiography can be applied after vital signs are stable [1].

For patients with oral secretions, if there is no respiratory tract obstruction, it is recommended to complete tracheal intubation followed by closed airway suctioning.

If repeated intubation is not successful and the patient's blood oxygen saturation is extremely low, it is recommended to quickly place the laryngeal mask for mechanical ventilation. After the oxygenation is improved, tracheal intubation will be reattempted.

5.3.7 Post-intubation Management

Improve Relevant Doctor's Prescription and Intubation Records.

Routine sedation is recommended to avoid collapse or even prolapse of tracheal tubes due to biting from restless patients. To avoid secondary intubation caused by prolapse of tracheal tube, if necessary, muscle relaxants can be used to eliminate spontaneous breathing, and a nursing doctor's advice on tracheal intubation should be prepared with the use of 0.5% erythromycin ointment to protect the cornea.

Lung protective ventilation strategy, i.e., mechanical ventilation with low tidal volume (4–8 mL/kg, ideal body weight) and low inspiratory pressure (plateau pressure <30 cm H_2O) to reduce ventilator-associated lung injury, and arterial blood gas can be checked for adjustment of respiratory parameters [5].

5.3.8 Post-intubation Sedation and Analgesia Plan for Patients in Wards

Recommended regimen of sedation for intubated patients on ventilators:

1. Phase 1: Basic Sedation (overlay of one or two regimens as appropriate)
   (a) Pump infusion of Propofol 0.5~3.0 mg/(kg·h), increase or decrease as appropriate [6].
   (b) Pump infusion of Dexmedetomidine 0.2~1.4 μg/(kg·h), increase or decrease as appropriate [6, 7].
   (c) Pump infusion of Midazolam 0.02~0.1 mg/(kg·h), increase or decrease as appropriate [7].
2. Phase 2: Sedation + Analgesia (choose one as appropriate)
   (a) Pump infusion of Sufentanil 0.1~1 μg/(kg·h), increase or decrease as appropriate.
   (b) Pump infusion of Remifentanil 0.05~2.0 μg/(kg·min), increase or decrease as appropriate.
3. Phase 3: Sedation + Analgesia + Muscle Relaxation
   (a) Pump infusion of Rocuronium 0.01~0.012 mg/(kg·min), or single intravenous injection of Rocuronium 0.1~0.2 mg/kg.

5.4 Tracheotomy

Xiaomeng Zhang

For severe and critical COVID-19 patients, tracheal intubation and mechanical ventilation are major treatments to maintain their vital signs. However, tracheotomy should be considered if prolonged tracheal intubation could not effectively promote the drainage and suctioning of sputum, and it may seriously affect the airway patency of the patient and can cause ventilator withdrawal.

During tracheotomy, the splashing of airway secretions caused by opening of airway-related wound, cough reflex, and ventilator ventilation may spray the virus-carrying secretions upon medical personnel and form the massive aerosol into the surgical environment, thus greatly increasing the risk of nosocomial dissemination [8]. Therefore, the primary task during tracheotomy is to protect the medical staff and the surgical environment from nosocomial infection.

Usually, percutaneous dilation tracheotomy should be preferred. It is a minimally invasive surgical method with the advantages of less time-consuming, less splashing, and operable at bedside [9]. However, some patients are not suitable for percutaneous dilation tracheotomy due to their neck conditions. At this point, traditional tracheotomy is an inevitable choice, though it is more dangerous than percutaneous tracheotomy.

5.4.1 Preoperative Evaluation

For patients undergoing elective tracheotomy, orotracheal intubation and mechanical ventilation are usually performed. Custodians, anesthesiologists, and otolaryngologists should conduct a comprehensive pre-surgery assessment to choose the appropriate timing and mode of tracheotomy. Whether early tracheotomy after mechanical ventilation with intubation facilitates early withdrawal of ventilator is still under academic controversy [10]. However, it is a consensus among all disciplines that the removal of tracheal intubation through the mouth can increase the comfort of the patient. Sedatives can be discontinued or reduced as soon as possible, and the replacement of tracheal intubation with tracheotomy, would reduce respiratory dead space and work of breathing. Therefore, upon comprehensive multidisciplinary assessment, elective tracheotomy may be generally considered when extubation cannot be performed after more than 7 days of orotracheal intubation and conventional mechanical ventilation, or in a short period of time. For those who are not suitable for percutaneous dilation tracheotomy mainly due to short neck, thyroid hyperplasia, cervical scar contracture, etc., traditional tracheotomy may be considered.

5.4.2 Mode of Anesthesia

Since most of the COVID-19 patients are scheduled for elective tracheotomy, it is recommended to perform tracheotomy under general anesthesia after tracheal intubation from a safe prospective.

For very few COVID-19 patients with upper airway obstruction who require emergency tracheotomy, surgery should be performed after tracheal intubation under general anesthesia. If it has to be done under local anesthesia, it is necessary to prepare for intubation under general anesthesia at the same time.

5.4.3 Preoperative Preparation

Preparation of personal protective equipment: It shall be carried out according to Level III protection criteria, including protective suits, N95 masks, goggles, foot covers, gloves, and positive pressure ventilation head covers.

Preparation of surgical environment and instruments: in consideration of the limited vision and operation of the operator under Level III protection criteria, except for the percutaneous dilation tracheotomy, all traditional tracheotomy should be carried out in the operating room with good lighting, suction devices, energy surgical instruments such as an electric knife or bipolar electrocoagulation in place, so as to reduce bleeding and obtain a clear operation vision.

Preparation of operating personnel: a group of three operators is recommended, among which one is the main surgeon, one the assistant, and the third can work as a back-up person to replace the one with discomfort at any time.

Preparation of anesthesia personnel: Preoperative assessment before general anesthesia and preparation for tracheal intubation under general anesthesia, control of anesthesia machine during surgery, replacement of intubation by mouth with ventilation through tracheostomy tube, etc.

5.4.4 Surgical Indications

Secretion retention caused by severe COVID-19 in the lower respiratory tract.

COVID-19 complicated with other diseases (such as stroke, postcranial surgery, thoracoabdominal trauma, and myasthenia gravis) resulting in weak cough or inability to cough, who require long-term orotracheal intubation after evaluation.

Those with upper airway obstruction combined with novel coronavirus infection: severe laryngeal obstruction caused by laryngeal inflammation, tumors, trauma, or foreign bodies.

5.4.5 Relative Surgical Contraindications

Critical COVID-19 patients are often associated with severe coagulation abnormalities and thrombocytopenia. Operation should be carried out after the correction and improvement of these conditions.

Surgery can be performed after correction and improvement of the severe anemia.

5.4.6 Absolute Surgical Contraindications

1. Patients with tension pneumothorax
2. Hypovolemic shock
3. Patients with heart failure, especially right heart failure
4. Patients with bullae, pneumothorax, or pneumomediastinum without drainage
5. Patients with massive hemoptysis
6. Patients with recent acute myocardial infarction

5.4.7 Surgical Precautions

Follow the procedures of the tracheotomy with the same surgical risks and precautions. For traditional tracheotomy in COVID-19 patients, the surgeon should communicate and cooperate with the anesthesiologist, paying special attention to avoid splashing of airway secretions during tracheotomy, so as to avoid increasing the exposure risk for medical personnel and aerosol formation in the surgical environment. Specific measures may include ventilation through machine and totally stopping spontaneous respiration during surgery, avoiding pinching the balloon when incising the anterior wall of trachea, and transient cessation of mechanical ventilation from the timing of trachea incision to cannula insertion.

5.4.8 Surgical Complications

Postoperative bleeding; wound infection; subcutaneous emphysema; pneumothorax and mediastinal emphysema; cannula prolapse; respiratory arrest; tracheoesophageal fistula; laryngotracheal stenosis; difficult extubation; rare complications, including innominate artery and common carotid artery injury, recurrent laryngeal nerve paralysis.

5.5 ECMO Support

Zhaohui Fu

According to the pathological characteristics of diffuse alveolar injury caused by acute inflammation of COVID-19, for severe patients with respiratory failure, if the protective ventilation strategy and prone position cannot effectively improve oxygenation and eliminate carbon dioxide, early ECMO treatment should be pursued in case of no contraindications to prevent the increase of transpulmonary pressure due to respiratory distress and inappropriate mechanical ventilation, avoid further aggravation of lung injury, reduce pulmonary and systemic inflammatory response, and prevent secondary extrapulmonary tissue and organ injury caused by severe long-term hypoxia, so as to help patients survive the acute phase, and create conditions and buy time for the recovery of lungs.

Precautions for the application of ECMO in COVID-19: Timing and mode of intervention, anticoagulation and bleeding, coordination with mechanical ventilation, early rehabilitation training, withdrawal criteria, and treatment of complications.

5.5.1 Timing of ECMO Intervention

When protective mechanical ventilation with low tidal volume is used, positive end-expiratory pressure (PEEP) $\geq$10 cm H_2O should be pursued combined with recruitment maneuver, prone position ventilation, neuromuscular block, and sedation. ECMO treatment is recommended when the following conditions occur with pure oxygen inhalation:

1. $PaO_2/FiO_2 < 100$ mmHg, or alveolar–arterial oxygen pressure difference [P (A-a) O_2] > 600 mmHg.
2. Ventilation frequency <35 breaths/min, pH < 7.2.
3. Plateau pressure >30 cm H_2O.
4. Age <65 years old.
5. Duration of mechanical ventilation <7 days.
6. No contraindications: Irreversible primary disease; severe brain dysfunction; anticoagulant contraindications; advanced age >80 years; BMI > 45 kg/m^2; high

ventilatory support level [airway plateau pressure >30 cm H_2O, FiO_2 > 0.8] applied for more than 7~10 days. However, ECMO has no absolute contraindications. It is crucial to weigh the pros and cons and communication with the patient's family for decision making.

7. The condition is potentially reversible.

5.5.2 Establishment of ECMO

Since the risk of blood splashing during the establishment of ECMO for COVID-19 patients is high, and due to the operational inconveniences possibly caused by multiple protections, in order to establish ECMO tubing as quick and accurate as possible and minimize infection, the following suggestions for the operation and protection during the establishment of ECMO are proposed:

1. Prepare 800 mL of suspended red blood cells, 400 mL of plasma, and 40 g of 20% human albumin in case to correct hypovolemia, coagulation function, and platelet count before catheterization.
2. The goggles must undergo sufficient antifogging treatment, so as to avoid affecting the visual field during operation.
3. Patients need adequate sedation and analgesia to prevent accidental body movement during operation, which will result in unnecessary tissue damage and prolonged operation time.
4. If possible, Level III protection can be applied.
5. Bedside ultrasound must be used to assess vascular conditions, cardiopulmonary function, and hemodynamic status before puncture.
6. Use ultrasound to measure the inner diameter of target puncture vessel, and correctly select the model of catheter. The inner diameter of catheter should not exceed 2/3 of that of the vessel.
7. Catheterization should be guided in real time using ultrasound localization.
8. Prepare for incision and catheterization. For patients with poor vascular conditions and failed puncture, multiple attempts should not be made to prevent severe vascular injury and massive hemorrhage.
9. After catheterization, the position of the drainage tube should be assessed ultrasonically before securing the catheter. The femoral drainage tube should be placed at the entrance of the vein into the right atrium.

5.5.3 Mode Selection

V-V mode should be applied for patients with simple respiratory failure, and V-A mode should not be preferred for possible circulatory problems;

For patients with respiratory failure who have cardiogenic shock due to a combination of severe cardiovascular dysfunctions (PaO_2/FiO_2 < 100 mmHg), V-A-V mode should be selected, and maintain V/A = 0.5/0.5 by limiting flow; since

COVID-19 patients have severe pulmonary lesions and may have progressive aggravation of pulmonary conditions during ECMO, it is not recommended to use VA-ECMO to provide respiratory and circulatory support at the same time.

For COVID-19 patients without severe respiratory failure who have cardiogenic shock due to a combination of severe cardiovascular events, V-A mode should be selected for ECMO support, but mechanical ventilation will also be needed and awake ECMO should be avoided.

Given that COVID-19 patients treated with ECMO suffer from multiple organ dysfunctions, and medical and nursing personnel are in extreme shortage, ECMO treatments when patients' conscious is clear are not recommended.

5.5.4 Flow Setting and Target of Oxygen Supply

The initial flow shall be >80% of CO (cardiac output).

$SPO_2 > 90\%$ and $FiO_2 < 0.5$ should be maintained during the maintenance.

Initial airflow regulation in V-V mode: blood flow: airflow = 1:1, basic target: $PaCO_2 < 45$ mmHg;

Be alert to the dysfunction of membrane lung caused by the accumulation of condensate due to long-term low airflow. It is necessary to regularly and intermittently increase the airflow to reduce the accumulation of condensate.

HCT should be maintained at 40–45% to ensure oxygen supply.

In the initial stage, sedation and analgesia or even muscle relaxant can be administered to avoid fever and tachycardia as well as reduce oxygen consumption.

Assess volume status to ensure normal cardiac output.

5.5.5 Setting of Ventilation Target

After ECMO operation, $FiO_2 < 0.5$ can be pursued, respiratory rate can be reduced by 4–10 breaths/min, and appropriate PEEP of 10–15 cm H_2O can be applied. According to respiratory mechanics monitoring, super protective mechanical ventilation (VT < 4 mL/kg) should be applied to make driving pressure <10 cm H_2O and plateau pressure <25 cm H_2O.

Prone position ventilation, lasting >12 h/day, can be administered during ECMO to promote lung recruitment. Be alert to unplanned extubation, catheter displacement, tube entanglement, pressure sore, etc. Reassess the position of catheter ultrasonically after prone position ventilation ends.

5.5.6 Anticoagulation and Bleeding Prevention

Before catheterization, for patients without active bleeding or visceral bleeding and platelets >80 × 109/L, the first loading dose of 20–30 U/kg is recommended.

For patients with a combination of bleeding risk or platelet <50 × 109/L, component transfusion should be performed before catheterization to increase platelet count to be above 80 × 109/L and correct FiO_2—4 g/L; coagulation PT should not be prolonged longer than 3–5 s against normal value; AT III should be maintained above 80%.

Coagulation function or ACT should be monitored every 4 h. The anticoagulation dose target can be maintained as APTT (activated prothrombin time) 60–80 s, or ACT 160–200 s, with reference to the trend of D-dimer; if possible, thromboelastography should be monitored intermittently.

In case of ECMO with heparin-free anticoagulation, for the purpose of getting active bleeding or fatal bleeding under control, where ECMO support cannot be discontinued, the all-heparin coated circuit and catheter with blood flow >3 L/min may be considered for heparin-free operation with recommended operation time <24 h, and equipment and consumables for replacement should be prepared in advance; anticoagulation should be gradually restored once active bleeding ceases or coagulation improves.

During heparin anticoagulation, if APTT cannot be up to standard and coagulation occurs, antithrombin III (ATIII) activity should be monitored. If activity reduces, fresh frozen plasma should be supplemented to restore heparin sensitivity.

As for heparin-induced thrombocytopenia (HIT), immune-mediated production of heparin platelet factor 4 (PF4) antibodies is present in patients, which results in abnormal platelet aggregation and thrombosis. Argatroban may be used as a substitute.

Attention should be paid to bleeding or exudation in the catheterization site, alimentary tract, invasive operation site, and intracranial area. The anticoagulation intensity can be reduced or anticoagulation can be suspended altogether depending on the severity of the bleeding event; if anticoagulation is discontinued, attention should be paid to the possibility of thrombosis in the catheter and membrane lungs, and a readily available ECMO system should be prepared at the bedside for replacement. Antifibrinolytic therapy can be used for treating surgical bleeding.

Thromboelastography should be monitored carefully to obtain a complete picture of coagulation and fibril volume.

Avoid unnecessary invasive procedures as much as possible to reduce bleeding.

5.5.7 Catheter-Related Bloodstream Infections

The majority of COVID-19 patients require prolonged VV-ECMO support, with prevention of blood flow in related catheters being a top priority. If possible, treatment should be carried out in a single room with special care by designated medical personnel. In patients with ECMO support for more than 1 week, PCT and CRP should be closely monitored, and attention should be paid to the sudden increase of body temperature or no increase in body temperature. In patients with ECMO support for over 2 weeks, regular blood cultures and G tests are recommended, so as to monitor bloodstream infections. During the process of ECMO withdrawal, blood cultures, and cultures from intravascular catheter tips should be obtained. In addition to Gram-positive bacteria, Gram-negative bacteria should not be ignored in the bloodstream infections of ECMO patients either, most of which are multiple or pan-resistant bacterial infections, such as CRAB and CRE.

During administration of antibiotics, attention should be paid to the lipid solubility of the drug, protein binding rate and the patient's heart, liver and renal function, as well as serum albumin level, while adjusting the dosage and monitoring the drug concentration if possible.

5.5.8 ECMO Withdrawal

When the etiology is eliminated or condition improves, tidal volume recovery and CO_2 removal capacity are improved under the same support conditions, the ventilator should be maintained as follows before ECMO withdrawal:

1. Inhaled oxygen concentration <50%.
2. Tidal volume is 6–8 mL/kg, airway plateau pressure <25 cm H_2O, PEEP $\leq$ 10 cm H_2O.

Under the above conditions, blood flow of ECMO shall be lowered to 2 L/min without changing ECMO oxygen concentration, and observe it for 24 h. If vital signs are stable, experimental withdrawal could be considered. When lowering the flow, pay attention to strengthen anticoagulation so as to avoid thrombosis.

Experimental withdrawal: Blood flow of VV-ECMO and anticoagulation will remain unchanged with airflow of ECMO being turned off; changes in SaO_2, $PaCO_2$, airway pressure, respiratory rate, tidal volume, etc. will be monitored; duration of monitoring: 2–4 h. In case of SaO_2 > 95% and $PaCO_2$ < 50 mmHg, ECMO withdrawal may be considered.

References

1. Chen X, Liu Y, Gong Y, Guo X, Zuo M, Li J, Shi W, Li H, Xu X, Mi W, Huang Y. Chinese Society of Anesthesiology CAoA: perioperative management of patients infected with the novel coronavirus: recommendation from the Joint Task Force of the Chinese Society of Anesthesiology and the Chinese Association of Anesthesiologists. Anesthesiology. 2020;132:1307–16.
2. Scott JA, Heard SO, Zayaruzny M, Walz JM. Airway management in critical illness: an update. Chest. 2020;157:877–87.
3. April MD, Arana A, Pallin DJ, Schauer SG, Fantegrossi A, Fernandez J, Maddry JK, Summers SM, Antonacci MA, Brown CA III, Investigators N. Emergency department intubation success with succinylcholine versus rocuronium: a National Emergency Airway Registry Study. Ann Emerg Med. 2018;72(6):645–53.
4. Ahmad I, El-Boghdadly K, Bhagrath R, Hodzovic I, McNarry AF, Mir F, O'Sullivan EP, Patel A, Stacey M, Vaughan D. Difficult Airway Society guidelines for awake tracheal intubation (ATI) in adults. Anaesthesia. 2020;75(4):509–28.

5. Meng L, Qiu H, Wan L, Ai Y, Xue Z, Guo Q, Deshpande R, Zhang L, Meng J, Tong C, Liu H, Xiong L. Intubation and ventilation amid the COVID-19 outbreak: Wuhan's experience. Anesthesiology. 2020;132:1317–32.
6. Xia ZQ, Chen SQ, Yao X, Xie CB, Wen SH, Liu KX. Clinical benefits of dexmedetomidine versus propofol in adult intensive care unit patients: a meta-analysis of randomized clinical trials. J Surg Res. 2013;185(2):833–43.
7. Riker RR, Shehabi Y, Bokesch PM, Ceraso D, Wisemandle W, Koura F, Whitten P, Margolis BD, Byrne DW, Ely EW, Rocha MG, Group SS. Dexmedetomidine vs midazolam for sedation of critically ill patients: a randomized trial. JAMA. 2009;301(5):489–99.
8. Tran K, Cimon K, Severn M, Pessoa-Silva CL, Conly J. Aerosol generating procedures and risk of transmission of acute respiratory infections to healthcare workers: a systematic review. PLoS One. 2012;7:e35797.
9. Margolin G, Ullman J, Karling J. A new technique for percutaneous tracheotomy. Otolaryngol Head Neck Surg. 2017;156:966–8.
10. Hosokawa K, Nishimura M, Egi M, Vincent J. Timing of tracheotomy in ICU patients: a systematic review of randomized controlled trials. Crit Care. 2015;19:424.

Special Diagnosis and Treatment for Patients with COVID-19

6

Yong Zhang, Yong Liu, Fang Zheng, Yu Zhang, Yuyong Su, Xuefeng Cai, Yong Gao, Rui Chen, and Jianchu Zhang

Contents

The corresponding author of Sect. 6.1 is Yong Zhang, Email: mailzhangyong@126.com
The corresponding author of Sect. 6.2 is FangZheng, Email: fangzheng99@sina.cn
The corresponding author of Sect. 6.3 is Yu Zhang, Email: whxhzy@163.com
The corresponding author of Sect. 6.4 is Yong Gao, Email: docgao@163.com
The corresponding author of Sect. 6.5 isYong Gao, Email: docgao@163.com
The corresponding author of Sect. 6.6 is Rui Chen, Email: unioncr@163.com
The corresponding author of Sect. 6.7 is Jianchu Zhang, Email: zsn0928@163.com

Y. Zhang (✉)
Department of Hepatobiliary Surgery, Union Hospital, Tongji Medical College, Huazhong University of Science and Technology, Wuhan, China

Y. Liu · Y. Gao
Department of Orthopaedics, Union Hospital, Tongji Medical College, Huazhong University of Science and Technology, Wuhan, China

F. Zheng
Department of Pediatrics, Union Hospital, Tongji Medical College, Huazhong University of Science and Technology, Wuhan, China

Y. Zhang · Y. Su · X. Cai
Department of Pharmacy, Union Hospital, Tongji Medical College of Huazhong University of Science and Technology, Wuhan, China

R. Chen
Department of Integrated Traditional Chinese Medicine and Western Medicine, Union Hospital, Tongji Medical College, Huazhong University of Science and Technology, Wuhan, China

J. Zhang
Department of Respiratory and Critical Care Medicine, Union Hospital, Tongji Medical College, Huazhong University of Science and Technology, Wuhan, China

F. Cheng, Y. Zhang (eds.), *The Clinical Diagnosis and Treatment for New Coronavirus Pneumonia*, https://doi.org/10.1007/978-981-15-5975-4_6

6.1 Emergency Surgery

6.1.1 Principle of Handling COVID-19 Complicated with Emergency Surgery

Yong Zhang

For the patients diagnosed with COVID-19 complicated with emergency surgery, medical staff, on the one hand, need to formulate individualized treatment protocols in a timely manner in strict accordance with the diagnosis and treatment principles of emergency surgery; on the other hand, they need to carry out COVID-19 screening and treatment,

All emergency surgical patients in need of observation or hospitalization are subject to routine tests, including CT scan of lungs, SARS-CoV-2 nucleic acid testing with nasopharyngeal swabs, IgM and IgG antibody detection and general laboratory tests. In addition to COVID-19 screening, relevant surgical workup is also required, such as B-mode ultrasound, radiography, and CT imaging evaluations. CT has a higher diagnostic value for surgical emergencies and can be completed simultaneously with the CT scan of lungs. The patients with higher possibility of surgery are recommended to receive relevant examinations at one time as early as possible, such as blood routine, blood biochemistry, coagulation function, pretransfusion examination, etc., to avoid increased risk of cross-infection due to multiple blood drawings. Vascular surgical acute abdomen mainly includes type B aortic dissection, abdominal aortic aneurysm, superior mesenteric artery dissection or thrombosis, and portal vein thrombosis. For the patients with acute abdomen due to vascular causes, aortic CTA and B-mode ultrasound of abdominal vessels must be performed in addition to other required routine surgical examinations.

Lung injury due to mechanical ventilation under anesthesia, surgical stress, postoperative pain, and difficulty in expectoration due to slow cough reflex may aggravate pulmonary inflammation or lead to the COVID-19 progression, especially for the patients with severe and critical COVID-19. However, in order to save lives in an emergency, the indications for emergency surgery must be fully controlled with adequate preparation and strict protection to avoid missing the best time for treatment. In addition to saving lives, reducing injury and protecting functions, surgeries must be designed with streamlined processes and shortened duration to avoid increasing the infection or exposure rate of medical staff. Preoperative discussions must be presided over by the doctors with associate senior titles or above, with the doctors on emergency duty from the surgery department, anesthesiology department, infectious disease department, operating room, etc. involved. Preoperative discussions may be done by telephone or video in the hospital to clarify the necessity of emergency surgery, anesthesia method, surgical approach and processes, possible problems and solutions [1].

Device preparation: The instruments, consumables, and drugs for surgeries should be prepared and placed in the operating room as much as possible depending on the type of surgery; the medical staff for surgeries should be designated and unrelated persons are not allowed for access; surgeries should be performed with disposable surgical kits, instruments, excipients, and consumables. For the patients with hemorrhagic surgical emergency, it is necessary to prepare sufficient blood for intraoperative use. The delivery personnel and channel are prepared in advance.

6.1.2 General Surgery (Including Vascular Surgery)

Yong Zhang

Acute abdomen in general surgery refers to rapid pathological changes in abdomen, pelvic cavity, retroperitoneal tissues, and organs, resulting in clinical syndromes mainly manifested as abdominal symptoms and signs accompanied by systemic reactions, which is a common disease in emergency surgery and requires timely and effective treatment.

6.1.2.1 Nonsurgical Treatment

Acute abdomen patients infected with COVID-19 do not need emergency surgery since they have stable vital signs, mild local symptoms, no peritonitis, or active bleeding, such as acute simple appendicitis, acute simple cholecystitis, incomplete intestinal obstruction, etc., can be considered for outpatient observation or hospitalization to receive nonsurgical medical treatment including fasting for solids and liquids, GI decompression, anti-inflammatory therapy and nutrition support, and receive close observation of the changes in their conditions. Temporary nonsurgical treatment may be considered for the abdominal aortic aneurysm patients with no significant abdominal pain or mild abdominal pain, tumor diameter <5 cm on CTA, and superior mesenteric artery dissection or thrombosis without peritonitis. Conservative treatment or interventional embolotherapy is preferred to the advanced liver cancer patients with ruptured hemorrhage and mild simple splenic injury.

6.1.2.2 Surgical Treatment

Surgical treatment should be considered if nonsurgical treatment fails and the condition is progressively aggravated. The patients with significant abdominal signs, even diffuse peritonitis or massive active bleeding, must immediately step into the processes of emergency surgery once the indications for emergency surgery has been confirmed.

Intraoperative protection: In case that emergency surgery is required to the patients with COVID-19, all the contacts shall enter the negative-pressure operating room via a specific channel following level III preventive measures. Emergency surgery must be finished in a rapid and effective manner to reduce the time of operation and exposure of medical staff as far as possible while relieving the source of the patient's disease. Excised surgical specimens should be directly placed in double-sealed specimen bags and immersed in the fixative in the operating room. The specimen bags should be marked with "COVID-19" and then placed at the specified position. Strict disinfection of operating room, devices, and anesthesia machines should be timely performed after the surgery. For the patients who cannot be ruled out from COVID-19, it is also necessary to take standard protective measures in postoperative recovery period, especially when removing laryngeal masks and transferring with higher risk of exposure and infection. During the transfer, it is necessary to take surgical and ward elevators to avoid contact between the patients and other personnel.

Selection of anesthesia methods: For the patients not infected with COVID-19, anesthesia methods can be selected by routine, while for the patients with suspected and confirmed COVID-19, the anesthesia methods can be selected according to the patient's condition, surgical method, and operation scale: ① For level-3 surgery such as appendectomy and repair of gastroduodenal perforation, epidural anesthesia can be applied for laparotomy, and the patient must wear a mask correctly during the anesthesia; ② For level-4 surgery such as colectomy, general anesthesia can be applied, during which a laryngeal mask is recommended to establish an artificial airway to avoid increased risk of infection due to a large amount of aerosol in lungs excreted from the body as the conventional tracheal tube penetrates into the airway. Anesthetists must wear masks when performing tracheal intubation or removing the catheter to prevent airway secretion ejection caused by patient coughing.

Selection of surgical methods: Laparotomy should be applied as much as possible, as laparoscopic surgery that requires intubation under general anesthesia will increase the risk of cross-infection caused by aerosol excretion from the lungs; in addition, CO_2 pneumoperitoneum established by laparoscopic surgery may carry body fluids out of the abdomen, increasing the risk of aerosol transmission in the confined operating room, which may lead to the infection of medical staff if there is any improper operation [2].

Emergency surgery of gallbladder and biliary tract:

Percutaneous gallbladder drainage under local anesthesia can be considered for patients with acute cholecystitis and gallbladder empyema who are in very poor physical condition and cannot tolerate surgery at all. If the drainage effect is poor and the infection is aggravated, laparotomy should be timely performed.

For patients who can tolerate anesthesia and surgery, open cholecystectomy and/or bile duct exploration are preferred, with basic surgical process same as that of regular surgeries. However, since being susceptible to the interference of visual field and sense of touch when taking level III protective measures, surgeons should try to identify the bile duct structure during the surgery; if it is difficult to dissect the Calot's triangle, partial cholecystectomy can be performed after gallstones are removed to avoid common bile duct injury.

The presence of gallstones in common bile duct should be carefully evaluated before and during the surgery to avoid omission. For patients in good pulmonary and general conditions with satisfactory anesthetic effect, intraoperative choledochoscopy is feasible, and a T tube should be placed after gallstone removal. For patients in critical condition who cannot tolerate a long period of surgery, the T tube can be placed for drainage immediately after the removal of most of gallstones. Potential intraoperative biliary problems should be considered for the patients with gallbladder diseases; it is still recommended to prepare the equipment and devices for bile duct exploration to reduce handling and time consumption.

For biliary obstruction caused by malignant tumors, PTCD is preferred. Surgical treatment can be considered in patients who fail to respond to conservative treatment and can benefit from choledochotomy and drainage after imaging evaluation.

Rupture hemorrhage of liver and spleen:

Blood loss and blood product consumption should be adequately assessed before the surgery to ensure a smooth channel for blood product delivery. Take preventive measures for blood splashing when opening the abdomen.

Since intraoperative vision is limited and operations are more difficult, the incision should be fully exposed, so as to find bleeding points as soon as possible for subsequent hemostasis.

Care should be taken to avoid omission or accidental injuries due to poor vision.

Type B aortic dissection and abdominal aortic aneurysm.

Minimally invasive endovascular surgery under local anesthesia + sedation: DSA-guided aortic endovascular stent-graft exclusion.

Superior mesenteric artery dissection or thrombosis.

Minimally invasive endovascular surgery under local anesthesia + sedation: DSA-guided superior mesenteric arteriography, and superior mesenteric artery stenting or catheter-directed thrombolysis according to the angiographic conditions [3, 4].

Postoperative treatment: Closely observe the condition and change of drainage tube after surgery, monitor the patient's body temperature, and regularly re-examine blood routine, procalcitonin, and C-reactive protein. Special attention should be paid to patients with fevers to timely identify the cause.

After surgery, patients with COVID-19 should receive simplified treatment as much as possible with efficacy guaranteed, so as to reduce the contact between doctors and patients and avoid cross infection; only 1 caregiver is allowed, the access control should be strict, and visiting should be declined. The patients and caregivers should be required to take protective measures (publicity and education, correct wearing of masks, daily body temperature measurement) and sign a COVID-19 informed consent form and a letter of commitment. As COVID-19 is mainly transmitted by droplets and contact, all the medical staff, patients, and their families must wear masks correctly, and medical staff should take level III protective measures in strict accordance with the protection requirements when performing a short-distance operation or invasive operation. For patients inserted with nasal cannulas for oxygen inhalation or gastric tubes, appropriate masks should be selected to completely cover their mouths and noses as far as possible. Positive viral nucleic acid can be detected in the feces of patients with COVID-19, suggesting that COVID-19 may be transmitted by fecal–oral route. Therefore, disposable items, vomitus, feces, and drain fluid of patients with suspected or confirmed COVID-19 should be placed in double-sealed yellow garbage bags labeled as "COVID-19", and then disposed as infectious medical wastes. Medical staffs and caregivers exposed to the patients with COVID-19 should be subjected to medical observation for 14 days in principle, and receive timely treatment in case of any discomfort.

6.1.3 Orthopedic Trauma

Yong Liu

COVID-19 has spread the world since December 2019 and now has become a pandemic [5, 6]. COVID-19 patients could develop other conditions such as orthopedic disease. For instance, those elderly, especially those with chronic diseases, are more likely to develop serious orthopedic diseases. In this special outbreak, hospitalization for regular orthopedic patients should be avoided in general to decrease the risk of transmission, but operations are still necessary for some of them. This chapter shares some experience in the diagnosis and treatment of COVID-19 patients with traumatic and orthopedic disease.

First, people with chronic orthopedic diseases are not recommended for surgical treatment generally if the symptoms are not severe and bearable, such as lumbar disc herniation, femoral head necrosis. In those situations, selective surgery is preferable [7, 8]. The COVID-19 virus can directly damage the lungs, and cause inflammatory storms, attack lymphocytes that cause immune deficiency. As a result, the risk of surgery will increase, and surgeries become will be a huge threat to life. Therefore, we do not recommend surgery during the spread of COVID-19. However, we could treat pneumonia first until nucleic acid test becomes negative, symptoms like fever and cough disappear, IgG antibody is positive. After a further 14 days of quarantine after discharge, the patient could be admitted to the non-COVID-19 designated hospital after a repeat nucleic acid test and chest CT. Patients can be admitted and prepared for surgery only when the repeat tests are normal.

However, some patients may suffer from severe and even life-threatening disorders, such as fast-growing tumors not suitable for radiotherapy and chemotherapy, spinal cord compression in spinal stenosis which caused respiration difficulty and cauda equina syndrome, and acute joint infection which may cause shock. Under those circumstances, the symptoms could gradually develop and may lead to serious complications if proper surgery is not timely performed. For these patients, we should have a joint consultation with anesthesiologists, respiratory doctors and ICU doctors, and try our best to guarantee the safety of their lives. Moreover, minimal-invasive surgery is highly recommended, and the duration of operation should be shortened as much as possible. After the COVID-19 is cured, a second stage of operation could be further considered if needed.

If an emergency relevant to orthopedic disease occurred, conservative treatment is the first choice. For example, for those patients suffering from closed fractures without obvious vascular and nerve injury, we should try to choose noninvasive, rapid, and effective techniques such as close reduction, brace fixation, closed reduction external fixation, or homeopathic traction external fixation for fracture fixation. These strategies could restore limb length, correct deformity, achieve the purpose of reducing the patient's pain. At the same time, try to satisfy the following three points: (1) Correct fracture deformity and maintain the basic counterpoint of fracture end; (2) Reduce the patient's pain as much as possible and avoid obvious psychological discomfort; (3) Ensure a relatively stable fixation of the fracture end. For patients with active bleeding at the fracture end or who are over 65 years old and in poor physical condition, or patients with fracture types such as stable fractures of pelvis, supportive treatment should be included such as blood transfusion and so on.

During COVID-19's bursting, emergent surgery is applicable to patients suffering from unstable vital sign, gradually developing symptoms and injuries so as to save life and body function, such as patients with open fractures combined with vessel and nerve injury, open reeducation for a major joint dislocation patient after a failed close reduction, unstable vertebrate fracture with developing spinal cord injury symptoms or even respiratory dysfunction caused by high-level cervical fracture. It is necessary to improve the relevant examination. In addition, before surgery, multiple departments such as respiratory department, intensive care unit, and anesthesiology department should coordinate the consultation to assess the patient's physical condition and surgical risk with surgeons. As lifesaving comes first, minimal-invasive and short-time surgery is also the first choice for surgeons when selecting the operation methods. Second stage surgeries to improve body functions such as internal fixation could be performed after the COVID-19 is cured. The anti-coagulant treatments are needed while with great caution for patients with active bleeding. In addition, activities of lower limbs should be encouraged to prevent deep venous thrombosis of lower limbs.

At last, we would like to make a notice that some lab tests are very important for doctors to predict the prognosis of the patients before and after surgery. As studies have indicated that plasma cytokine storm was associated with pulmonary inflammation such as IL-6, TNF-α, and so on [9]. Those cytokines such as IL-6 could further target immune cells such as regulatory T cells (Treg) [10]. As a result, patients are more vulnerable to poor prognosis. In our hand, we performed four surgeries on COVID-19 patients until now. Three patients recovered well, with relatively normal Il-6 level and lymphocyte counts before and after surgery (detail of one case at the end of the chapter). However, one old man aged 80 years died of acute respiratory dysfunction. He developed 50-fold increment of Il-6 level and a dramatic 60% decrease of lymphocyte counts after surgery. Although the invasive ventilation and various supportive treatments were performed, he passed away 9 days post surgery. Therefore, we greatly suggest that doctors should regularly check lymphocyte numbers, lymphocyte subgroups, and serum cytokines, especially IL-6 level. If there is an obvious abnormality of those results, doctors must pay very close attention and try to intervene as early as possible.

A Successful Case of Surgery on COVID-19 Patient with Thoracolumbar Fracture

On February 18, 2020, a patient with COVID-19 complicated with thoracolumbar fracture and incomplete paralysis was transferred to Wuhan Union Hospital. He initially presented to Wuhan Hanyang District Hospital after a convulsive episode and found himself unable to move lower extremities after that. The patient reported that when he was resting on the sofa on the day of initial presentation, he suddenly developed convulsion with teeth clenching and limb shaking, but symptoms resolved spontaneously after a few seconds. When he was trying to get up, he noticed back pain and was unable to move his lower limbs. He sought medical attention at Wuhan Hanyang District Hospital and was hospitalized, underwent Magnetic resonance image of thoracolumbar spine which showed 12th thoracic vertebra burst fractures, first lumbar vertebral compression fractures. Incidentally on the CT, it showed bilateral pulmonary exudative changes, indicating a possible COVID-19 infection.

On February 17, 2020, the patient developed a cough without fever, and throat swab nucleic acid test turned out to be positive later. There was also no improvement in his paralysis after conservative treatment in that hospital. Subsequently, he was transferred to the Wuhan Union Hospital for COVID-19 treatment.

At the time of presentation to Wuhan Union Hospital, the patient had stable vital signs, with body temperature 36.6 °C, blood pressure of 124/86 mm Hg, pulse rate 87/min, breathing rate 16/min, oxygen saturation 98% in ambient air and normal mentation. Physical examination revealed bilateral lungs coarse breath sounds with some rales. There was tenderness in the thoracolumbar spine, hyperalgesia below the level of bilateral groin area with left side more severely involved, preserved cremasteric reflex, no saddle anesthesia, and normal anal sphincter tone. As for muscle strength: bilateral flexion hip strength 1/5, left ankle dorsiflexion and toe extensor muscle 2/5, right ankle dorsiflexion, and toe extensor muscle strength 2+/5. The bilateral knee tendon reflexes and Achilles tendon reflexes were reduced, and pathological reflexes were not elicited. Both ASIA and Frankel's spinal cord injuries were grade C per guideline.

From day 2 to day 9 of hospitalization, the patient's vital signs remained stable, afebrile and pulse oximetry remained above 97%, cough also improved slightly. His hospitalization was complicated by the left common iliac vein thrombosis identified by venous duplex, for which an inferior vena cava filter was placed before the orthopedic surgery.

On February 22, 2020, the patient underwent surgery with posterior open reduction and pedicle screw internal fixation of thoracolumbar fracture with standard three-level protection of all personnel in the operation room. In the morning, a physician wearing level two personal protective equipment (PPE) transported the patient from quarantine ward to the entrance of the operating room, then the anesthesiologist and operating room nurse took over. After successful general anesthesia, the surgeon upgraded PPE from level 2 to level 3. The C-arm was used to locate the injured vertebra, followed by incision of the skin and subcutaneous fascia, kyphotic deformity of T12 and L1 was seen. Screws and longitudinal rod were placed from T11 to L2 and retracted, with the kyphosis deformity resolved. The incision was rinsed with saline multiple times, and vancomycin was evenly sprinkled on the incision. After surgery, patient was transferred to ICU for recovery from general anesthesia. The whole operation lasted 2 hours and 43 min.

On post operation day 1, the patient was transferred from ICU back to the general quarantine ward. His vital signs remained stable, afebrile. Anti-inflammatory and analgesic medications were given. There were no signs of infection or abscess formation around the wound. Spinal cord function was evaluated on Post-op day 3: The hyperalgesia of both lower limbs was significantly alleviated, muscle strength gradually improved to 4/5, he could almost stand up with some assistance 3 weeks after surgery.

During the postoperative period, to understand the 2019nCoV, we checked patients' lymphocyte subsets, plasma cytokines, and 2019-nCoV antibodies. On the 3rd, 6th, and 14th day after the operation, the 2019-nCoV nucleic acid test was all negative, his cough resolved, remained afebrile, and an oxygen saturation of 98%. Repeat CT of thoracolumbar spine revealed that the lung exudation was absorbed, and the spinal reduction appeared satisfactory. He was discharged 3 weeks after surgery.

6.2 Pediatric Diagnosis and Treatment

Fang Zheng

Based on the existing epidemiological data, the incubation period of SARS-CoV-2 infection in children is between 1 and 14 days, mostly ranging from 3 to 7 days. It has been reported that the present data supports the possibility of maternal–fetal transmission [11]. Ninety percent of children have relatively mild clinical manifestations, without fever or pneumonia, and mostly recover within 1–2 weeks [12].

6.2.1 Diagnosis [13, 14]

Suspected case: Those with 1 epidemiological history plus 2 clinical manifestations.

Confirmed case: Suspected cases with one of the etiological diagnosis items.

Clinical classifications: There are five types of COVID-19 based on severity, including asymptomatic infection, acute upper respiratory tract infection, mild pneumonia, severe pneumonia, and critical cases, see Table 6.1.

6.2.2 Differential Diagnosis

It is mainly differentiated from other pathogen infections.

6.2.3 Treatment

The principle of treatment in children is the same as that of COVID-19 in adults, but the following matters should be paid attention to during the treatment of children:

6.2.3.1 Symptomatic Treatment

Acetaminophen and ibuprofen are recommended to control the active hyperpyrexia at the appropriate dosage, but should not be used in combination. Aspirin is not recommended as antipyretics. For patients with increased airway secretions, expectorants can be taken orally or by aerosol inhalation to dilute secretions to facilitate coughing up. Antitussive drugs should be used with caution. For patients with diarrhea, fluid replacement, probiotics, intestinal mucosal protective agents, and zinc supplementation should be given as supportive treatment, but antidiarrheal drugs should be used with caution.

Table 6.1 Clinical types of COVID-19 in children

Evaluation item	Asymptomatic infection	Acute upper respiratory tract Infection	Mild pneumonia	Severe pneumonia
General condition	Good	Good	Good	Poor
Consciousness disturbance	No	No	No	Yes
Hypoxemia	No	No	No	Cyanosis; shortness of breath: <2 months of age, respiratory rate (RR) ≥60 times/min; 2–12 months of age, RR ≥50 times/min; 1–5 years of age, RR ≥40 times/min; >5 years of age, RR ≥30 times/min, except for the effects of fever and crying Assisted respiration (moaning, flaring nares, three concave sign) Intermittent apnea Oxygen saturation < 92%
Fever	No	Severe case criteria not met	Severe case criteria not met	Hyperthermia for ≥5 days
Dehydration signs/apastia	No	No	No	Yes
Chest CT	No	No	Severe case criteria not met	Bilateral pulmonary infiltrates or multilobar infiltrates, with rapid progression within 24–48 h, or pleural effusion
Extrapulmonary complications	No	No	No	Yes
Diagnostic criteria	All of the above	All of the above	All of the above	Any of the above

Note: Critical and severe cases meet one of the following conditions: ① respiratory failure, requiring mechanical ventilation; ② shock; ③ combined with organ failure of other systems, needing admission to PICU for treatment

6.2.3.2 Antiviral Therapy

There is no specific antiviral drug. At present, interferon α spray or aerosol inhalant is recommended; since the efficacy of anti-influenza drugs including Abidol and Oseltamivir remains to be clarified, attention should be paid to their adverse reactions such as nausea, diarrhea, elevated liver enzyme and bradycardia during trial.

6.2.3.3 Antibacterial Drugs

Avoid mindless or inappropriate use, especially in combination with broad-spectrum antibacterial drugs, chloramphenicol, tetracyclines, sulfonamides, and aminoglycoside antibiotics should be avoided. For patients with liver and renal function impairment, the dose should be adjusted according to the degree of impairment.

6.2.3.4 Immunotherapy

Glucocorticoids can be used for a short period of time (3–5 days) for severe and critical cases at a recommended dose not exceeding the equivalent of 1–2 mg/(kg.d) of methylprednisolone; human immunoglobulin may be considered as appropriate, but the efficacy still needs further evaluation.

6.2.3.5 Treatment of Neonatal Critical and Severe Cases [15]

Effective organ function supportive therapy is performed on the basis of symptomatic treatment. For children in critical condition manifesting as "white lung", high-dose pulmonary surfactant, nitric oxide inhalation, and high-frequency oscillatory ventilation may be effective; glucocorticoids should be used with caution; 2 g/kg of gamma globulin should be administered in divided doses; CRRT and ECMO can be performed if necessary.

6.3 Rational Use of Antibacterial Drugs

Yu Zhang, Yuyong Su and Xuefeng Cai

Viral infection can cause serious damage to respiratory defense mechanism, weaken the bacterial clearance ability of the body, thus easily leading to secondary bacterial infection. It has been reported [16] that the majority of COVID-19 patients received antibacterial therapy [16]. How to avoid blindly or inappropriately using antibiotics is of crucial importance.

6.3.1 Strictly Grasps the Indications for Antibiotics Usage to Avoid Blindly or Inappropriately Using [17]

In general, antibiotics are not used for mild and moderate patients.

Moderate patients may develop into a severe condition due to any of the following factors: (1) persistent high fever; (2) advanced in years (over 60 years old); (3) with severe underlying diseases; (4) significant progression of lesions >50% within 24–48 h on pulmonary images; and (5) immunosuppressed individuals. Such patients need to be checked for the infection indicators such as white blood cell (WBC), neutrophil percentage, C-reactive protein (CRP) and procalcitonin (PCT) in hemogram and evaluated for possible etiology. If there is no evidence of infection, do not prescribe antibiotics and instead of dynamically observing the changes of infection indicators.

For moderate patients who may develop into severe type, it is necessary to identify whether there are risk factors for drug-resistant bacterial infection (out-of-hospital use of broad-spectrum antibacterial drugs for at least 3 days, structural lung disease, and positive culture of drug-resistant bacteria in airway secretions). In the absence of the above risk factors, it is recommended to select β-lactams + macrolides or respiratory fluoroquinolones alone according to the Guidelines for the Diagnosis and Treatment of Adult Community Acquired Pneumonia in China (2016 Edition) [18]. Empirical use of the antibacterial drugs for special use such as glycopeptides, carbapenems, and oxazolidinones is not recommended; if necessary, there should be laboratory evidence of bacterial infection and a consultation for the antibacterial drugs for special use. Sputum smears for bacterial and fungal staining and cultures and blood G + GM tests should be rechecked in patients who experience recurrent, long-lasting course of disease, or persistent lymphopenia. Anti-aspergillus drugs may be taken if necessary.

For severe and critical patients [19, 20]: Routine prophylactic use of antibacterial drugs, especially in combination with broad-spectrum antibacterial drugs, is not recommended. Third-generation cephalosporins/enzyme inhibitor complexes may be used empirically in patients confirmed to be complicated with bacterial infections. For patients with disease course of more than 2 weeks or low lymphocyte count, the presence of bacterial infection cannot be assessed by procalcitonin (PCT) and C-reactive protein (CRP) alone. Comprehensive judgment should be made in combination with body temperature, white blood cell count (WBC), neutrophil percentage, pulmonary imaging, and oxygenation function.

For patients in critical condition subject to airway opening such as invasive mechanical ventilation or extracorporeal membrane oxygenation (ECMO): They are susceptible to bacterial infections and fungal infections at a later stage [19]. For patients with septic shock, antibacterial drugs can be used empirically in combination before obtaining the etiological diagnosis, covering the most common infections with Enterobacteriaceae bacteria, *Staphylococcus*, and *Enterococcus*. β-Lactamase inhibitor complexes can be applied for those who experience infection after hospitalization. In case the therapeutic effect is poor, or the patient has severe septic shock, carbapenems can be used instead. If combined with enterococcal or staphylococcal infections are considered, empirical treatment with glycopeptides may be performed, and oxazolidinones can be applied if pulmonary infections are predominant. Catheter-related infections should be highly emphasized, methicillin-resistant *Staphylococcus* should be empirically covered for treatment, and glycopeptides can be selected for empirical treatment. Since some patients in critical condition often experience secondary fungal infections in the late stage, triazoles or echinocandin antifungal drugs can be used, but the combination of the two antifungal drugs is not recommended.

6.3.2 Identify the Pathogen of Secondary Infection as Early as Possible, and Select Antibacterial Drugs According to the Pathogen Types and Drug Sensitivity Test Results

Before the administration of antibacterial drugs, reasonable etiological examination and specimen sampling should be arranged for hospitalized patients to identify the pathogen and drug sensitivity results as soon as possible. When the etiological examination yields a significant positive result, target therapy (de-escalation therapy) should be performed [18, 21]. Drug sensitivity test of outpatients should be performed based on their conditions.

Before no pathogen and drug sensitivity results are obtained, initial antimicrobial therapy should be empirically performed according to the place of onset, primary lesion, age, underlying disease, clinical characteristics, laboratory and imaging examinations, disease severity, liver and renal functions, previous medications, possible pathogens, and drug resistance risk factors of patients.

Attention should be paid to the patient's history of antibacterial drug use, and the assessment of the effect of previous medications can assist in the identification of infectious pathogens [22].

Molecular biological techniques such as high-throughput sequencing, which can improve the sensitivity of pathogen detection and shorten the detection time, can be prudently used for etiological detection of secondary infections according to the situation of medical institutions [21].

After obtaining the results of pathogen detection, colonized bacteria should be distinguished from pathogenic bacteria according to the patient's condition and therapeutic effect to assess the significance of positive pathogen culture [21, 23, 24].

6.3.3 Develop an Antibacterial Drug Treatment Plan in Combination with Patient's Condition, Types of Pathogens, and Characteristics of Antibacterial Drugs

The appropriate dose of antibacterial drugs should be selected according to the site of COVID-19 secondary infection. For severe infections (sepsis, infective endocarditis, etc.), the antibacterial drugs should be given at a larger dose; while for secondary urinary tract infections, the drugs should be given at a lower dose.

The administration times of antibacterial drugs should refer to their PK/PD characteristics [25]. For time-dependent antibacterial drugs (such as penicillins, cephalosporins, monocyclic β-lactams, and carbapenems), better clinical efficacy can be achieved by multiple doses per day according to the half-life. Concentration-dependent antibacterial drugs (such as aminoglycosides, quinolones) are usually administered once a day.

The administration method of antibacterial drugs should follow the WHO medication principle of "drugs that may be taken orally shall not be administered by intramuscular injection, and drugs that may be administered by intramuscular injection shall not be done by infusion." For patients with mild secondary bacterial infection, oral anti-infective drugs with higher bioavailability should be selected as far as possible.

Laboratory test results and the response to initial antibacterial therapy should be timely reassessed after the administration of antibacterial drugs, continuation of antibacterial therapy or adjustment of antibacterial therapy regimen will be determined based on the assessment results.

During the treatment, attention should be paid to the identification of the source of secondary infection, which should be removed in time. For example, the catheter should be timely removed in case of catheter-related bloodstream infection, and urinary catheter should be timely removed in case of urinary catheter-related urinary tract infection.

6.4 Anti-Interleukin-6 Antibody Therapy

Yong Gao

Cytokine storm, such as typically with interleukin 6 (IL-6) elevations, is an important cause of death in COVID-19 patients in critical and severe conditions. Thus, antagonism of IL-6 elevation and inhibition of the generation of inflammatory factor storm become an important method for the COVID-19 treatment in critical and severe patients. Tocilizumab is a recombinant humanized anti-human IL-6 receptor monoclonal antibody currently used to treat adult patients with moderate-to-severe active rheumatoid arthritis who have had an inadequate response to disease-modifying antirheumatic drugs. Therefore, tocilizumab is expected to treat COVID-19 patients in critical condition.

6.4.1 Evaluating Indications for Medication [26–29]

6.4.1.1 Applicable Population

(a) Patients confirmed with moderate NCP (including high-risk factors for severe cases) and severe NCP
(b) Patients aged 18–85 years
(c) Patients with elevated IL-6 (recommended to be tested by Roche electrochemiluminescence)

Note: Moderate NCP (including high-risk factors for severe cases): Moderate NCP with bilateral pulmonary multiple lesions, or significant progression of lesions showed on pulmonary images >50% within 24–48 h.

6.4.1.2 Non-applicable Population

(a) Pregnant or lactating women
(b) Patients with ALT/AST >5 times ULN, neutrophils $<0.5 \times 10^9$/L, platelets $<50 \times 10^9$/L
(c) Patients confirmed with rheumatoid immune disease, malignant tumors, and other related diseases

(d) Patients orally taking antirejection drugs or immunomodulatory drugs for a long time
(e) Patients allergic to tocilizumab or any of the excipients
(f) Patients with active hepatitis and tuberculosis complicated with definite bacterial infection and fungal infection
(g) Organ transplant patients
(h) Patients with mental disorders

6.4.2 Signing the Informed Consent Form

Informed consent form must be signed by all patients before receiving anti-human IL-6 receptor monoclonal antibody treatment.

6.4.3 Use of TocilizumabDosing Regimen [26–29]

The initial dose is 4–8 mg/kg. The recommended subsequent dose is 400 mg into100 ml of normal saline for infusion over 1 h. For febrile patients, it continues to be febrile after usage within 24 h, a second dose with the same dosage can be applied at an interval ≥ 12 h; the maximum number of cumulative doses is twice, and the maximum single dose is no more than 800 mg.

6.5 Convalescent Plasma Therapy

Yong Gao

Convalescent plasma therapy [30–34] is a very effective and important method for severe and critical cases. Convalescent plasma therapy has been included in the fifth edition of the Diagnosis and Treatment Plan, and further refined in the sixth and seventh edition of the plan. Convalescent plasma therapy refers to reduce the virus content in patients by virus-specific antibodies of a certain titer in the plasma of survivors, so as to achieve the anticipated therapeutical purpose. At present, the treatment of existing cases has shown good efficacy in clinical practice. The convalescent plasma is subject to strict quality control requirements from its collection, preparation, and storage to clinical application.

6.5.1 Collection

COVID-19 survivors who voluntarily donate plasma should not only meet the common health requirements for voluntary blood donation, but also follow the corresponding procedures, and meet the criteria for release from isolation and discharge in the *COVID-19 Diagnosis and Treatment Plan (Version 6)*:

Collecting subjects: Post recovery and discharge >14 days, no fever or other medical history, no history of hazard exposure or close contact within 14 days; age 18–55 years; male weight > 50 kg, female weight > 45 kg; glucocorticoid withdrawal ≥1 week; interval from the previous plasma collection >14 days; no blood-borne diseases; being able to donate plasma as assessed by clinicians.

Collection method: Single collection; 200–400 mL of plasma is collected from a donor each time according to the donor's own willingness as determined by clinicians evaluation; the medical staff should closely observe the conditions of donors on the spot. In case of adverse reactions, the reactions will be timely prevented and treated according to the conditions on the spot.

Post-collection test: In addition to general quality test and the tests related to blood-borne diseases, plasma samples should also be submitted for test:

1. Single-sample detection of SARS-CoV-2 nucleic acid: negative.
2. It is recommended that the IgG antibody titer in SARS-CoV-2 serum should be no less than 160. The virus neutralization test can be applied, or the sample should be diluted by negative plasma by 160 times before testing to determine the total antibody level.

6.5.2 Clinical Indications of Convalescent Plasma Therapy

It is suitable for COVID-19 patients in severe and critical conditions with rapid disease progression and disease course of less than 7 days as follows:

1. Age ≥ 18 years.
2. COVID-19 patients confirmed by PCR, with positive nucleic acid within 48 h after plasma therapy.
3. Rapid disease progression or clinical indications conforming to severe case criteria.
4. Critical and severe patients must also meet the following:
   (a) Mechanical ventilation < = 48 h.
   (b) Creatinine clearance >50 Ml/min; ALT/AST <2× upper limit of normal; cTNI <2× upper limit of normal.
   (c) IL-6 and/or IL-2 < 2× upper limit of normal.

6.5.3 Inappropriate Clinical Indications

1. Patients who refuse to sign the informed consent for plasma therapy.
2. Patients under the age of 18 years.
3. Pregnant and lactating women.
4. Patients with the history of allergy to plasma infusion, sodium citrate, methylene blue, and immunoglobulin.
5. Patients with the history of autoimmune diseases and selective IgA deficiency.

6. Patients with severe underlying diseases.
7. In areas where conditions permit, high-titer COVID-19-RBD antibodies can be detected.

6.5.4 Infusion Dose

Usually, 100–500 mL (4–5 mL/kg body weight) of infusion may be given once or in two divided doses, depending on the clinical condition, the patient's weight, etc.

6.5.5 Principle of Infusion

Blood type: The blood of the same type (ABO) is preferred, followed by the blood of compatible types.

Infusion rate: Slowly first and then faster, no more than 20 drops/min in the first 15 min. If there is no discomfort, the infusion can be adjusted to the normal rate. Observe closely during the infusion; suspend or stop the infusion if any adverse reactions occur.

6.6 Traditional Chinese Medicine

Rui Chen

6.6.1 Period, Pattern, and Syndrome Differentiation

According to the COVID-19 Diagnosis and Treatment Plan (Trial Version 7) [35] issued by the National Health Commission of the People's Republic of China, COVID-19 can be divided into the cases in medical observation period and the cases in clinical treatment period. The cases in the medical observation period refer to preventive or suspected cases, which are divided into the cases with predominance of wetness and predominance of heat; while the cases in the clinical treatment period referring to confirmed cases, are divided into mild, moderate, severe, critical, and convalescence cases based on syndrome differentiation. Mild cases are divided into cold-damp constraint in the lung pattern and damp-heat accumulation in the lung pattern, moderate cases into damp-toxin constraint in the lung pattern, and cold-damp obstructing the lung pattern, severe cases into epidemic toxin blocking the lung pattern and blazing of both *qi* and *ying* pattern. Critical cases only refer to internal blockage and external desertion pattern, and convalescence cases are divided into *lung–spleen* deficient *qi* pattern and *qi-yin* deficiency pattern.

6.6.2 Pattern Identification and Treatment

Cases with predominance of wetness in medical observation period: It mainly manifests as fatigue with gastrointestinal discomfort, which should be treated with *Huoxiang Zhengqi oral liquid.*

Cases with predominance of heat in medical observation period: It mainly manifests as fatigue with fever, which should be treated with *Lianhuaqingwen* capsules.

Universal formula in clinical treatment period: It is applicable to the diagnosed patients at all stages; they can be treated with No. 1 formula of the Wuhan Union Hospital (West Campus) which is same as the *QingfeiPaiduGranule* (Decoction), if their syndromes cannot be timely differentiated.

Cold-damp constraint in the lung pattern of mild cases in clinical treatment period: It mainly manifests as fever, poor appetite, loose stool, pale enlarged tongue with white, thick and greasy coating, which should be treated with No. 2 formula of the Wuhan Union Hospital (West Campus) combined with *Maxing Yigan* Decoction, *Dayuan* Decoction, and Peptic Powder.

Damp-heat accumulation in the lung pattern of mild cases in clinical treatment period: It mainly manifests as fever, sore throat, muscle pain, nausea, and light red tongue with thin and yellow coating, which should be treated with No. 5 formula of the Wuhan Union Hospital (West Campus), i.e., *JinqiangXuanfeiJiedu* Mixture.

Damp-toxin constraint in the lung pattern of moderate cases in clinical treatment period: It mainly manifests as fever, chest tightness, and distressed cough with little sputum, constipation, dark-red, and enlarged tongue with yellow greasy or dry coating, which should be treated with the No. 1 formula of Wuhan Union Hospital (West Campus) at double dose.

Cold-damp obstructing the lung pattern of moderate cases in clinical treatment period: It mainly manifests as low fever, fatigue, stuffy feeling in chest, vomiting, loose stool, and pale tongue with white and greasy coating, which should be treated with the No. 2 formula of Wuhan Union Hospital (West Campus) at double dose.

Severe toxin lung-blocking pattern in clinical treatment period: It mainly manifests as fever, cough with little sputum or blood-stained sputum, tachypnea and short of breath, constipation, and red tongue with yellow and greasy coating, which should be treated with the No. 3 formula of Wuhan Union Hospital (West Campus) composed of *Maxingshigan* Decoction, *HuopuXialing* Decoction, *raw rhubarb, astragali radix, semen lepidii*, and *red paeony root.*

Blazing of both *qi* and *ying* pattern of severe cases in clinical treatment period: It mainly manifests as high fever, polydipsia, tachypnea, unconsciousness, bleeding or convulsion, and crimson tongue with little coating, which should be treated with *Baihu* Decoction combined with *ShuiniujiaoDihuang* Decoction.

Internal blockage and external desertion pattern of critical and severe cases in clinical treatment period: Mechanically ventilated patients, mainly manifested as unconsciousness, sweating, cold extremities; the pulse is floating and large without root; the patients should be treated by taking *Storax* Pills or *AngongNiuhuang* Pills with the No. 6 formula (*Ginseng* 15 g, *Radix AconitiPraeparata* 10 g, *Cornus officinalis* 15 g) of Wuhan Union Hospital (West Campus). In case of constipation or patient-ventilator asynchrony, dissolve 10 g of *Raw Rhubarb* powder with warm water for intragastric administration.

Lung–spleen qi deficiency pattern of convalescence cases in clinical treatment period: It mainly manifests as shortness of breath, fatigue, poor appetite, loose stool, and pale tongue with white coating during convalescence, which should be treated with the No. 4 formula of Wuhan Union Hospital (West Campus), combined with *XiangshaLiujunzi* Decoction.

Qi-yin deficiency pattern of convalescence cases in clinical treatment period: It mainly manifests as shortness of breath, fatigue, dry mouth, dry cough, and red tongue with scant liquid, which should be treated with *WuyeLugen* Decoction or 50 ml of warm water diluted *Shengmai* injection for oral use.

The above formulas and decoctions are selected according to the corresponding patterns, 1 dose per day, decocted in water for oral dose, 2–4 times a day, 100–200 ml each time according to the condition.

6.6.3 Use of Chinese Patent Medicine Injection

Viral infection or complicated with mild bacterial infection: 0.9% sodium chloride 250 ml plus *Xiyanping* injection 100 mg, bid, or 0.9% sodium chloride 250 ml plus *Reduning* injection 20 ml, or 0.9% sodium chloride 250 ml plus *Tanreqing* injection 40 ml, bid.

High fever with altered mental status: 0.9% sodium chloride injection 250 ml plus *Xingnaojing* injection 20 ml, bid.

Systemic inflammatory response syndrome or/and multiple organ failure: 0.9% sodium chloride injection 250 ml plus *Xuebijing* injection 100 ml, bid.

Weakness and dry mouth: *Shenmai* Injection 100 ml, bid, or *Shengmai* Injection 20–60 ml, bid.

Shock and cold extremities: 0.9% sodium chloride injection 250 ml plus *Shenfu* injection 100 ml, bid; when shock occurs, 50 ml *Shenfu* injection can also be pumped.

6.6.4 Precautions for Use of Chinese Patent Medicines

1. Generally, among the same type of Chinese patent medicine injections, only one is used.
2. Traditional Chinese medicine injections can be used in combination with traditional Chinese medicine decoctions, capsules, and granules.
3. Since *Xuebijing* injection has a risk of bleeding, it should be used with caution when there is a tendency to bleed.
4. Only *Shenfu* injection should be used in shock, and Chinese patent medicines such as *Xiyanping* and *Tanreqing* should not be used in combination.

5. If it has been determined that the allergy, liver and renal dysfunction are caused by the traditional Chinese medicine, please discontinue the drug in time and provide with symptomatic treatment.
6. The use of traditional Chinese medicine injections should follow the package insert and the principle of starting from a small dose and gradually adjusting based on syndrome differentiation.

6.6.5 Typical Cases Treated with the Combination of Traditional Chinese Medicine and Western Medicine

Mr. Zhu, male, 69 years old. W8 West Ward 41.

He complained of "fever and cough for 12 days" and was admitted to the hospital on February 10, 2020, with "COVID-19." At the time of TCM intervention, he had been hospitalized for 7 days and had an onset of 19 days.

History of present illness: The patient had fever, cough, and other symptoms without obvious etiology12 days ago, with the Tmax of 39.2 °C. Then, the cough was progressively aggravated without temperature change, accompanying with coughing, and a small amount of blood-stained sputum. No obvious fatigue, chest distress, nasal congestion, shortness of breath, sore throat, diarrhea, abdominal distension, abdominal pain, urination discomfort, etc. The patient visited the Wuhan Union Hospital, and was given oral antiviral drugs after relevant examinations. After that, the symptoms were not improved markedly. The cough was aggravated recently and dyspnea was observed. On February 5, CT showed bilateral pulmonary multiple diffused thin patchy shadows. Infection was taken into consideration, not excluding viral pneumonia. Nucleic acid testing showed double positive. He was admitted to our hospital with diagnosis of "COVID-19."

Past medical history: Denied any history of chronic diseases.

Treatment process: After admission, he received western medicine treatment, including oxygen therapy, ribavirin antiviral therapy, meropenem antibacterial therapy, methylprednisolone anti-inflammatory therapy, *Xuebijing* treatment of systemic inflammatory response, and nutrition support therapy. However, with the respiratory support gradually increasing, the improvement was not significant. Assisted ventilation with a small noninvasive ventilator for home use was applied before TCM treatment, IPAP20cmH2O, EPAP4cmH2O, FiO2 80%. ECG monitoring: HR90 bpm, SpO2 92%, R25 times/min, Bp130/70 mmHg.

Current symptoms: Alert but low spirit, shortness of breath, dry mouth, no fever, stool once every 2–3 days, yellow urine, dark red tongue with yellow, thick and dry coating, and slippery and rapid pulse.

After TCM consultation, it was considered that damp-heat epidemic toxin and sputum stasis are stagnated in the lungs, which was planned to be treated with *HuayuJieDu* Decoction (No.3 formula of Wuhan Union Hospital, West Campus) at 3 doses, one dose per day; it was decocted in water, and take 500 ml of warm liquid for intragastric administration at five times, 100 ml each time.

Subsequent visit on February 20: After the medication for 2 days, cough and suffocation were improved, with respiratory support gradually reduced. Relevant re-examination situation as this given in figures. The tongue was slightly dark red with yellow and thick coating significantly improved, and the pulse was rapid. Take another 3 doses. The administration method we same as before.

Subsequent visit on February 23: The patient stated that the symptoms were relieved, yet SpO2 was 94%. Recently, the doctor of western medicine suggested to adopt intubation assisted ventilation instead for many times since it was difficult to reduce the ventilator support; the doctor of traditional Chinese medicine suggested suspending since the patient complained that the symptoms were relieved, who found that the dark red tongue was slightly aggravated while the coating was improved. The patient continued to take another 3 doses of *HuayuJiedu* Decoction.

Subsequent visit on February 26: The patient reported that the symptoms were relieved, which was most obvious after the administration of traditional Chinese medicine, SpO2 was 99%, and the support of ventilator was downregulated. The doctor of Western medicine canceled the suggestion of intubation assisted ventilation, and then the patient took the *HuayuJiedu* Decoction for more than half a month. By March 20, the patient's shortness of breath and chest distress were significantly improved, and nasal cannula oxygen administration was used instead, with SpO2 being 99%. Then the formula was changed to No.4 formula (convalescence) of Wuhan Union Hospital (West Campus) for body conditioning.

6.7 Bronchoscopy

Jianchu Zhang

Bronchoscopy has unique advantages in respiratory infectious diseases and in assisting airway management of critical patients. However, as COVID-19 has become a respiratory infectious disease of global concern, bronchoscopic diagnosis and treatment of such disease must follow strictly isolation and protection standards to reduce the risk of infection for medical staff. Therefore, bronchoscopy is not recommended as a routine examination for 2019-nCoV viral sampling [36]. As summarized from what we have conducted bronchoscopy during diagnosis and treatment, bronchoscopy has the following values in the diagnosis and treatment of COVID-19 patients:

1. Assist in the establishment of artificial airways and guide tracheal intubation or percutaneous tracheotomy.
2. Assist to manage the artificial airways, including sputum suction, removal of blood scab, and relief of airway obstruction.
3. Obtain samples from the lower respiratory tract to improve the positive rate of PCR testing and the accuracy of pathogen culture, and to reasonably guide the use of antibacterial drugs.
4. Assist in local treatment via bronchoscope with infusion of α-interferon and N-acetylcysteine.

Requirements for the personal protection and in the operation room: (1) When medical staffs operate bronchoscopy during diagnosis and treatment for COVID-19 patients, they are recommended to wear positive-pressure hoods in addition to level III protective measures [37]; (2) We should conduct the bronchoscopy in negative pressure wards as much as possible. For those without such conditions, it is recommended to provide well-ventilated separate rooms where are preferably equipped with air disinfectors of good performance.

In case the bronchoscopy is proposed to COVID-19 patients, medical staff should fully consider whether the patient has the indications and contraindications for the procedure, as well as the purpose and necessity of the procedure. However, the patients with established artificial airway have relatively few contraindications for the procedure. In the following cases, it is necessary to operate gently with caution to reduce the relevant complications during the procedure: (1) extremely unstable vital signs; (2) platelet count $<20 \times 10^9$/L; the procedure also can be performed after platelet transfusion; (3) malignant arrhythmia, unstable angina pectoris, and hypertensive crisis; (4) intracranial hypertension, etc.

Bronchoscope selection [38]: In order to reduce the risk of infection for medical staff during the procedure, avoid the influence of protective articles on visual field. Portable bronchoscopes or disposable bronchoscopes with display screens should be selected.

Specimen collection: (1) For COVID-19 patients who have not established artificial airway, bronchoscopy is not recommended as a routine operation for infection sampling; (2) For COVID-19 patients with established artificial airway, bronchial secretion, or bronchoalveolar lavage fluid samples can be obtained by bronchoscopy, thus to monitor the load of SARS-CoV-2 and examine whether it is complicated with bacterial, fungal, and other viral infections, assisting to guide clinical medications. There is no guideline for bronchoalveolar lavage in COVID-19 patients. Severe imbalance of ventilation/perfusion ratio (V/Q) is found in critical patients. So a large amount of bronchoalveolar lavage may lead to further aggravation of hypoxia or spread of infection. With reference to the *Chinese Expert Consensus on Pathogen Detection of Bronchoalveolar Lavage in Pulmonary Infectious Diseases* (2017 Edition) [39], the total amount of lavage is 60–120 ml (20 ml each time). (3) Specimens are stored and submitted for testing: Specimens should be submitted on ice as soon as possible after collection; they should be stored at room temperature for ≤30 min, at 4 °C for ≤4 h, and at −70 °C for >4 h. Sealed specimens should be placed in transfer boxes for infectious virus samples loaded with dry ice for transport by specially assigned person, to ensure that the specimens are still covered with dry ice when delivered to the testing institution (to prevent the degradation of RNA virus) [40].

For COVID-19 patients with established artificial airway, the requirements of anesthesia and ventilator setting for bronchoscopic diagnosis and treatment are as follows: (1) sedation and analgesia: In order to avoid aerosol generation caused by patient coughing and reduce the damage to the airway during operation, deep sedation, and muscle relaxant when necessary, may be given to the patients to improve patient–ventilator asynchrony; (2) ventilator setting during operation: (1) select volume-controlled ventilation (VCV or V-A/C); (2) PEEP: PEEP needs to be reduced to 6 cm H_2O, or be turned off when necessary; (3) FiO_2: set as 100%.

References

1. Jianing Y, Weiguo F. Suggestions on orderly vascular surgeries at all levels under the epidemic situation of novel coronavirus pneumonia. Chin J Gen Surg. 2020;35(3):E003.
2. Wang W, Jianhua H. Consideration and suggestions on diagnosis and treatment in vascular surgery under the epidemic situation of novel coronavirus pneumonia [J]. Chin J Gen Surg. 2020;29(02):137–41.
3. Kaixiong T, Bixiang Z, Peng Z, Zhu P, Wang G, Xiaoping C. Recommendations for general surgery clinical practice in 2019 coronavirus disease situation. Chin J Surg. 2020;58(03):E001.
4. Dalong Y, Lianxin L. Management strategy of prevention and control for surgeons to asymptomatic 2019-nCoV RNA positive corona virus diseases 2019 (COVID-19) [J]. Chin J Pract Surg. 2020;40(03):248–9.
5. Wang Z, et al. Clinical features of 69 cases with coronavirus disease 2019 in Wuhan, China. Clin Infect Dis. 2020:ciaa272.
6. Guo Y, et al. COVID-19 pandemic: global epidemiological trends and China's subsequent preparedness and responses. Zhonghua Liu Xing Bing Xue Za Zhi. 2020;41(5):643–8.
7. Guidelines on diagnosis and treatment of novel coronavirus pneumonia (trial sixth edition). Chin J Infect Control. 2020;19(02):192–5.
8. Liu J, Li H, Zhou W, et al. Expert consensus on emergency surgery management for traumatic orthopedics under prevention and control of novel coronavirus pneumonia. Chin J Trauma. 2020;36(02):111–116.5.
9. Wong CK, et al. Plasma inflammatory cytokines and chemokines in severe acute respiratory syndrome. Clin Exp Immunol. 2004;136(1):95–103.
10. Mahmud-Al-Rafat A, et al. Decoding the enigma of antiviral crisis: does one target molecule regulate all? Cytokine. 2019;115:13–23.
11. Dong L, Tian J, He S, et al. Possible vertical transmission of SARS-CoV-2 from an infected mother to her newborn. JAMA. 2020;323(18):1846–8. https://doi.org/10.1001/jama.2020.4621.
12. Dong Y, Mo X, Hu Y, et al. Epidemiological characteristics of 2143 pediatric patients with 2019 coronavirus disease in China. Pediatrics. 2020;145(6):e20200702. https://doi.org/10.1542/peds.2020-0702.
13. Chen Z, Fu J, Shu Q, et al. Diagnosis and treatment recommendations for pediatric respiratory infection caused by the 2019 novel coronavirus. World J Pediatr. 2020; https://doi.org/10.1007/s12519-020-00345-5.
14. Yi J, Lu X, Runming J, et al. Diagnosis, treatment and prevention of 2019 novel coronavirus infection in children: experts' consensus statement (second edition). Chin J Appl Clin Pediatr. 2020;35(2):143–9.
15. Working Group for the Prevention and Control of Neonatal 2019-nCoV Infection in the Perinatal Period of the Editorial Committee of Chinese Journal of Contemporary Pediatrics. Perinatal and neonatal management plan for prevention and control of SARS-CoV-2 infection (2nd edition). Chin J Contemp Pediatr. 2020;22(3):195–200.
16. Huang C, Wang Y, Li X, et al. Clinical features of patients infected with 2019 novel coronavirus in Wuhan, China. Lancet. 2020;395(10223):497–506. https://doi.org/10.1016/S0140-6736(20)30183-5.
17. General Office of the National Health Commission. Notice on issuing a COVID-19 diagnosis and treatment plan (Trial Version 7) (GWBYH [2020] No.145). http://www.nhc.gov.cn/yzygj/s7653p/202003/46c9294a7dfe4cef80dc7f5912eb1989.shtml.
18. Chinese Thoracic Society, Chinese Medical Association. Guidelines for the diagnosis and treatment of adult community acquired pneumonia in China (2016 edition). Chin J Tuberc Respir Dis. 2016;39(4):253–79.
19. Shanghai Clinical Treatment Expert Group for Corona Virus Disease 2019. Comprehensive treatment and management of corona virus disease 2019: expert consensus statement from

Shanghai. Chin J Infect Dis, 2020, 38 (2020-03-01). http://rs.yiigle.com/yufabiao/1183266.htm.DOI: https://doi.org/10.3760/cma.j.issn.1000-6680.2020.0016.
20. Chinese Research Hospital Association of Critical Care Medicine. Youth Committee of Chinese Research Hospital Association of Critical Care Medicine. Chinese experts consensus on diagnosis and treatment of severe and critical new coronavirus pneumonia. Chin Crit Care Med, 2020, 32 (2020-02-22). http://rs.yiigle.com/yufabiao/1182606.htm. DOI:https://doi.org/10.3760/cma.j.cn121430-20200218-00001.
21. Subspecialty Group of Infectious Diseases, Chinese Thoracic Society, Chinese Medical Association. Chinese guidelines for the diagnosis and treatment of adults with hospital-acquired and ventilator associated pneumonia. Chin J Tuberc Respir Dis. 2018;41(4):255–80.
22. Wang L, Zhou W, Cao Y, et al. Characteristics of Stenotrophomonas maltophilia infection in children in Sichuan, China, from 2010 to 2017. Medicine. 2020;99(8):e19250. https://doi.org/10.1097/MD.0000000000019250.
23. Chen B, He L, Hu B, et al. Chinese expert consensus on diagnosis, treatment, prevention and control of Acinetobacter baumannii infection. Natl Med J China. 2012;92(2):76–85.
24. Zhou H, Li G, Zhuo C, et al. Chinese expert consensus on diagnosis, treatment, prevention and control of Stenotrophomonas maltophilia infection. Natl Med J China. 2013;93(16):1203–13.
25. Falcone M, Paul M, Tiseo G, et al. Considerations for the optimal management of antibiotic therapy in elderly patients. J Glob Antimicrob Resist. 2020; https://doi.org/10.1016/j.jgar.2020.02.022.
26. Yonggang Zhou, Binqing Fu, Xiaohu Zheng, et al. Aberrant pathogenic GM-CSF+ T cells and inflammatory $CD14^+CD16^+$ monocytes in severe pulmonary syndrome patients of a new coronavirus. BioRxiv preprint February 20, 2020. doi: https://doi.org/10.1101/2020.02.12.945576.
27. Channappanavar R, Perlman S. Pathogenic human coronavirus infections: causes and consequences of cytokine storm and immunopathology. Semin Immunopathol. 2017;39:529–39. https://doi.org/10.1007/s00281-017-0629-x.
28. Cui W, et al. Expression of lymphocytes and lymphocyte subsets in patients with severe acute respiratory syndrome. Clin Infect Dis. 2003;37:857–9. https://doi.org/10.1086/378587(2003).
29. Zumla A, Hui DS, Azhar EI, Memish ZA, Maeurer M. Reducing mortality from 2019-nCoV: host-directed therapies should be an option. Lancet. 2020;395(10224):E35–6. https://doi.org/10.1016/S0140-6736(20)30305-6.
30. Shen C, Wang Z, Zhao F, et al. Treatment of 5 critically ill patients with COVID-19 with convalescent plasma. JAMA. 2020;323(16):1582–9. https://doi.org/10.1001/jama.2020.4783.
31. Mair-Jenkins J, Saavedra-Campos M, Baillie JK, et al. The effectiveness of convalescent plasma and hyperimmune immunoglobulin for the treatment of severe acute respiratory infections of viral etiology: a systematic review and exploratory meta-analysis. J Infect Dis. 2015;211(1):80–90.
32. Y. Cheng,·R Wong,·Y O Y Soo,·W. S. Wong, et al. Use of convalescent plasma therapy in SARS patients in Hong Kong. Eur J Clin Microbiol Infect Dis (2005) 24: 44–46 DOI https://doi.org/10.1007/s10096-004-1271-9.
33. Burnouf T, Seghatchian J. Ebola virus convalescent blood products: where we are now and where we may need to go. Transfus Apher Sci. 2014;51(2):120–5.
34. Chen L, Xiong J, Bao L, Shi Y. Convalescent plasma as a potential therapy for COVID-19. Lancet Infect Dis. 2020;S1473-3099(20):30141–9.
35. National Health Commission of the People's Republic of China. COVID-19 diagnosis and treatment plan (Trial Version 7). 2020-03-04; http://www.satcm.gov.cn/d/file/p/2020/03-04/ddfd72721be1d510657c1cb0a42cb045.pdf##ce3e6945832a438eaae415350a8ce964.pdf
36. Group of Interventional Respiratory Medicine, Chinese Thoracic Society. Expert consensus for bronchoscopy during the epidemic of 2019 novel coronavirus infection (trial version). Chin J Tuberc Respir Dis. 2020;43(03):199–202.
37. Shuijiang C, Wu L, Difei C, et al. Analysis of bronchoscope-guided tracheal intubation in 12 cases with COVID-19 under the personal protective equipment with positive pressure protective hood. Chin J Tuberc Respir Dis. 2020;43:332–4.

38. Respiratory care committee of Chinese Thoracic Society. Expert consensus on preventing nosocomial transmission during respiratory care for critically ill patients infected by 2019 novel coronavirus pneumonia. Chin J Tuberc Respir Dis. 2020;43:288.
39. Chinese Thoracic Society, Chinese Medical Association. Chinese expert consensus on pathogen detection of bronchoalveolar lavage in pulmonary infectious diseases. Chin J Tuberc Respir Dis. 2017;40(8):578–83.
40. Respiratory & Critical Care Medicine Group, Chinese Thoracic Society, Chinese Medical Association. Recommendations for airway management in adult patients with severe COVID-19 (trial). Natl Med J China. 2020;100(10):729–37.

Special Clinical Care

7

Jian Luo

Contents

The corresponding author of Sects. 7.1–7.6 is Jian Luo, Email: ljwhhbcn@163.com

J. Luo (✉)
Department of Nursing, Union Hospital, Tongji Medical College, Huazhong University of Science and Technology, Wuhan, China

F. Cheng, Y. Zhang (eds.), *The Clinical Diagnosis and Treatment for New Coronavirus Pneumonia*, https://doi.org/10.1007/978-981-15-5975-4_7

7.1 Oxygen Therapy for Critically Ill Patients

Jian Luo

7.1.1 Closely Monitoring the Disease [1–3]

Monitoring patient's vital signs, especially the changes in consciousness, respiratory rate, oxygen saturation, etc.

Patient's symptoms such as cough, expectoration, chest tightness, dyspnea, and cyanosis. Should be surveyed, and blood gas analysis should be dynamically monitored. Severe cases of patients should be provided with oxygen by nasal cannula or facial mask and be assessed timely if relieved from respiratory distress and/or hypoxemia.

Oxygen therapy through high-flow nasal cannula (HFNC) or noninvasive mechanical ventilation: When respiratory distress and/or hypoxemia of the patients cannot be relieved after the patients receive standard oxygen therapy, high-flow nasal cannula or noninvasive ventilation can be considered. If it does not improve or even worsens in a short period of time (1–2 h), tracheal intubation and invasive mechanical ventilation shall be performed as soon as possible.

Invasive mechanical ventilation: Mechanical ventilation should be provided by lung protective ventilation strategy, i.e., low tidal volume (6–8 mL/kg ideal body weight) and low-level airway plateau pressure (P_{plat} 30 cm H_2O), so as to reduce ventilator-related lung injuries. While ensuring the airway plateau pressure of 35 cm H_2O, PEEP can be adopted appropriately. The airway should be kept humidified and warm. Long-time sedation should be avoided. Patients should be woken up early and lung rehabilitation treatment should be carried out. In the situation of patient–ventilator asynchrony, sedatives and muscle relaxants should be used timely. Sealed endotracheal suctioning should be carried out based on the condition of airway secretions. If necessary, bronchoscopy should be performed and corresponding treatment should be provided.

7.1.2 Care of Patients Receiving High-Flow Nasal Cannula

High-flow (maximum 60–80 L/min) gas with relatively constant inspiratory oxygen concentration (21–100%), temperature (31~37 °C), and humidity should be provided to the patients, and oxygen therapy is provided by nasal plug [2].

7.1.2.1 Indications

When respiratory distress and hypoxemia cannot be improved after oxygen is supplied by nasal cannula or mask, mild-moderate type I respiratory failure (100 mmHg $\leq FiO_2 <$ 300 mmHg), mild respiratory distress (RR > 24 times/min), no indication for emergent tracheal intubation, supporting ventilator removal and extubation.

7.1.2.2 Relative Contraindications

Severe type I respiratory failure (FiO_2 < 100 mmHg), ventilatory disorder (pH < 7.35), paradoxical breathing, poor airway protection ability, high risk of aspiration, unstable hemodynamics, multiple organ dysfunction syndrome (MODS), abnormal mental state, requiring vasoactive drugs, patients who cannot wear HFNC due to surgery on the face or the upper respiratory tract, severe nasal obstruction, HFNC intolerance.

7.1.2.3 Absolute Contraindications

Patients whose heart beat and breath suddenly stop, requiring emergent invasive ventilation; patients with weak spontaneous respiration; patients with extremely severe type I respiratory failure (FiO_2 < 60 mmHg); ventilatory disorder (pH < 7.25).

7.1.2.4 Clinical Operation

7.1.2.4.1 Temperature Setting

The initial temperature for patients without tracheotomy should be set at 31–34 °C and can be appropriately adjusted based on the comfortability and viscosity of sputum; the initial temperature for patients with tracheotomy should be set at 37 °C.

7.1.2.4.2 Flow Rate

The initial flow rate should be set at 35–45 L/min. Titrate the inhaled oxygen concentration to maintain the oxygen saturation above 93%. The flow rate and oxygen concentration should be dynamically adjusted according to the result of blood gas analysis.

7.1.2.4.3 Criteria for HFNC Removal

HFNC parameters should be gradually decreased after the primary disease is under control. If HFNC < 25 L/min FiO_2 < 30% can be reached, the therapy can be changed to oxygen supply by nasal cannula.

7.1.2.4.4 Precautions

(1) Before connection of the machine, the doctor should communicate with the patient, explaining the purpose of the treatment and obtaining consent from the patient. (2) Body position: Semi-reclining position is recommended. (3) Appropriate model of nasal plug should be used and nasal cannula smaller than 50% of the inner diameter of the nostril is recommended. Reduced pressure dressing should be applied first upon use and the tightness of the fixing strap for nasal plug should be adjusted appropriately to avoid device-related pressure injury on the facial skin [2]. (4) Patients who open their mouths for breathing should be instructed to breathe with mouth closed. If they cannot cooperate, the therapy can be switched to nasal mask. (5) Over-humidification and under-humidification should be avoided, character of gas secretions should be closely observed, and sputum suction should be carried out as needed. (6) Attention should be paid to water accumulation in the tubing. (7) Attention should be paid to observe the changes in vital signs, form of respiratory

movement, and blood gas analysis during usage to avoid delayed intubation. (8) Attention should be paid to adjust the tightness of the nasal plug. (9) Attention should be paid to various warnings during usage and their timely handling. (10) After treatment with HFNC (within 1~2 h), the efficacy and reactions should be closely monitored. The other supporting methods should be used if the following conditions occur continuously: unstable hemodynamics, obvious movement of auxiliary ventilator, deterioration of consciousness, RR > 35 times/min, $SpO_2 < 90\%$, large quantity of airway secretions, combined $PCO_2 > 45$ mmHg, pH < 7.35, etc. In such conditions, the doctor should be informed; consider stopping HFNC oxygen therapy and providing mechanical ventilation timely by tracheal intubation [3, 4].

7.1.3 Disposal of Secretions

Patients should wipe their saliva, nasal discharge, and sputum on their own or under the assistance of the nurse. The secretions should be wrapped and discarded into a closed disposable container prefilled with disinfectant containing 2500 mg/L of chlorine. For patients requiring mechanical suction, the sputum should be sucked into a collector prefilled with disinfectant containing 2500 mg/L of chlorine. If patients accidently spill excretions on the ground or surface of an object, gloves should be worn, and moisture absorption method (high-quality tissue is recommended) should be used first to remove visible contaminants and then 1000 mg/L effective chlorine containing disinfectant should be used to wipe for 30 min before wiping with clean water. Cleaned secretions should be centralized and disposed of as medical wastes.

7.2 Care of Patients Receiving Mechanical Ventilation

Jian Luo

7.2.1 Cooperation for Tracheal Intubation

The number of doctors and nurses required for ensuring the safety of the patients should be limited, and positive pressure headgear should be worn [4]. Before intubation, analgesia and sedation should be carried out, and muscle relaxation should be performed as needed. Meanwhile, hemodynamics should be monitored well. Within 30 min postoperation, staff movement in the room should be reduced, and continuous plasma air purification should be carried out for disinfection.

7.2.2 Management of Analgesia, Sedation, and Deliration

The objective of analgesia and sedation should be determined daily. Analgesia degree should be evaluated Q4h (CPOT) and sedation be evaluated Q2h (RASS/BISS).

The analgesics and sedatives should be adjusted accordingly. Pre-analgesia should be carried out before operation that specifically causes pain. CAM-ICU deliration screening should be carried out at each shift so as to identify positive patients as early as possible. Bundle strategy for prevention of deliration should be implemented: pain handle, minimize sedation, communication, sleep promotion, early activity, etc. [1, 3]. After sedative and analgesic drugs are administered, the effects, circulation, and breathing conditions should be closely observed and recorded regularly.

7.2.3 Prevention of VAP [1, 3, 5]

VAP prevention bundle should be implemented, including following the hand hygiene system; raising the bed head of the patient by 30~45° if not contraindicated; performing oral care every 4~6 h; using disposable saliva absorption toothbrush; maintaining cuff pressure at 25~30 cm H_2O and monitoring every 4 h; providing nutrient solutions by gastric tube and monitoring residual amount in the stomach every 4 h; evaluating if the machine can be removed every day; using flushable tracheal catheter to continuously suck secretions under the glottis at low negative pressure, with pumping by 10 mL syringe intermittently q1h~q2h; and adjusting the suction frequency based on the actual quantity of secretions on the cuff. For residues under the glottis, 10 mL syringe should be used to suck the secretions on the cuff and then immediately suck appropriate amount of disinfectant containing 2500 mg/L of chlorine. Then the needle cap should be connected, and the syringe should be placed into a sharps box. It is recommended to use disposable ventilator circuit. Conventional replacement is not recommended, and the circuit should be timely replaced in case of contamination. Heat moisture exchanger should be replaced every 5–7 days and should be immediately replaced in case of contamination or failure.

7.2.4 Aspiration of Sputum

Aspiration of sputum: Closed endotracheal suctioning and closed disposable sputum collection bag should be used to reduce aerosol and droplets. Pure oxygen should be provided for patients for 2 min pre- and post-aspiration of sputum, and the duration of aspiration should not exceed 15 s.

Collection of sputum specimen: sputum collection device with closed endotracheal suctioning tube should be used to reduce exposure to droplets.

Observation and record: Attention should be paid to the vital signs of the patients and the character, color, and quantity of sputum.

7.2.5 Disposal of Condensate Water of Ventilator Tube [2, 3, 6]

It is recommended to use ventilator tubelines with disposable double circuit through heating guide wire and automatic water filling humidification tank to reduce the generation of condensate water.

When the ventilator tubeline is provided with the water collection cup, the position of the ventilator tubeline should be kept lower than the artificial airway, and the water collection cup at the circuit end should be at the lowest position for the drainage of condensate water, which should be poured in time. Capped container should be prefilled with disinfectant containing 2500 mg/L of chlorine. Two people are needed to cooperate in transferring of the accumulated water within the tube into the capped container and then directly dumped into a cleaning machine whose temperature can reach 90 °C for automatic cleaning and disinfection.

Before pouring the condensate water, nursing staff shall be well protected. It is recommended to press the standby key of the ventilator to stop ventilation before pouring. Then directly disconnect the ventilator near the gas outlet end of the ventilator before pouring. The purpose is to avoid accidental splashing of condensate water, which will contaminate the nursing staff, or to avoid the condensate water from going back into the airway of the patient.

7.2.6 Prone Position Ventilation [1, 4, 7]

Preparation before turning over: Sedative and analgesic drugs should be used in accordance with the prescriptions; gastric retention should be evaluated and enteral nutrition should be stopped in advance; secretions in the mouth, nose, and airway should be cleaned; unnecessary venous access should be disconnected and catheter should be properly fixed; preventive anti-stress dressing should be used to protect the stressed skin; electrode slice should be replaced.

During turning over: At least five medical staff should cooperate, one staff in charge of the head, responsible for tracheal intubation and coordinating the turning action of others, and two staff members at each side of the patient. The patient should be placed at a lateral position first and then changed to prone position to make sure that the chest, hip, and knee joint fall on a polymer pad or soft pillow to avoid pressing. The head of the patient should be tilted to one side, and a U-shaped pad should be placed under the stressed side of the head so as to prevent the tracheal tube from being stressed. The upper limbs of the patient should be in parallel with the body or slightly abduced, with the forearms placed upward at the head side or downward at both sides of the body. The functional position should be maintained, and brachial plexus injury caused by ischemia due to stretching and squeezing should be avoided. The heart rate and oxygen saturation should be monitored during turning; catheters should be protected to prevent detaching.

After turning over: Instruments should be connected and infusion should be resumed; catheters should be properly fixed; body position should be adjusted every 2 h; the skin and blood supply at the stressed skin should be observed to avoid stress injury.

7.2.7 Prevention of Aspiration [1, 3]

Monitoring and care of gastric retention: Postpyloric feeding with feeding pump should be continued to reduce gastroesophageal reflux. If conditions allow, gastric motility and gastric retention should be evaluated by ultrasound. Conventional evaluation is not recommended for patients with good gastric emptying.

Gastric retention amount should be evaluated every 4 h: Refeed if gastric retention amount is less than 100 mL, and report to the doctor if the gastric retention amount is more than 100 mL before making any decision.

Prevention of aspiration during transfer: Nasal feeding should be stopped before transfer; residual amount in the stomach should be withdrawn. The stomach tube should be connected with negative pressure bag for drainage; during transfer, the bed head should be raised by 30°.

Prevention of aspiration for patients receiving nasal high-flow oxygen therapy: Inspection should be carried out every 4 h to avoid and timely handle over-humidification or under-humidification and water accumulation in the tubeline. Attention should be paid to coughing and aspiration caused by entry into airway by mistake. The nose plug should be maintained at a position higher than the machine and tubeline, and condensate water of the tubeline should be handled in a timely manner.

7.2.8 Prevention of Stress Ulcer, Gastrointestinal Bleeding, and ICU Acquired Weakness [3]

Early identification of population with high risk of stress ulcer: When mechanical ventilation ≥ 48 h, those receiving renal replacement therapy and those with liver disease, combination of multiple complications, high organ failure score, blood coagulation disorders, etc. are all population with a high risk of stress ulcer.

Enteral nutrition in the early stage (24–48 h after hospitalization).

The color of the gastric drainage should be closely observed; during enteral nutrition, contents in the stomach can be withdrawn to observe their color; attention should be paid to the occult blood test results and the color of stool.

In the early disease stage or stable disease stage, conscious patients should be instructed to actively carry out activities of extremities. Patients with disturbance of consciousness should be provided with passive movement to prevent muscular atrophy and muscular weakness.

7.3 Routine Management and Monitoring of ECMO

Jian Luo

ECMO perfusionist should manage, check, and record the following hourly: rotation speed, blood flow, oxygen flow, oxygen concentration, if temperature controller is rotating and flowing and setting as well as the actual temperature, if blood clots are developed in the membrane oxygenation, if tubing is twisted and stressed, if venous tubeline is shaking, if the urine of the patient turns red or dark brown.

Check and record the following at each shift: Catheterization depth, tubeline fixing condition, if interfaces are firm, water level of temperature controller, power supply of the machine, gas supply connection, check if there is oozing and swelling at the puncture site at each shift, measure the thigh circumference of both lower limbs, observe if there is swelling of the lower limb at the operation side, and observe peripheral perfusion, such as pulsation of dorsal pedal artery, skin temperature, and color. Function of ECMO oxygenator should be evaluated at each shift.

Anticoagulation management: The purpose of ECMO anticoagulation is to prevent thrombosis and reduce the risk of bleeding. Common anticoagulation method: heparin anticoagulation. During rotating and flowing, heparin sodium should be used for maintenance (4–30 U/kg/h), heparin should be continuously pumped in to maintain ACT at 180–200 s; the number of skin punctures should be minimized during anticoagulation. Procedures should be gentle and bleeding status should be closely observed.

7.3.1 Daily Monitoring

Blood gas analysis: Blood gas analysis should be performed once every 3 h after stabilization. PaO_2 should be maintained at 80–120 mmHg and $PaCO_2$ at 35–45 mmHg.

ACT: ACT should be monitored once every hour in the early stage, and once every 3–6 h after ACT stabilized [1].

Body temperature: Body temperature should be monitored once every 4 h and maintained at 36–37 °C to avoid the increase of oxygen consumption caused by high body temperature and disorder of coagulation mechanism and hemodynamics [1].

Blood pressure: The blood pressure during ECMO may be low, especially in the initial stage. MAP of 50–60 mmHg should be maintained during the operation of ECMO.

For urine volume, the excess water during ECMO should be excreted through the kidney if possible. Urine volume should be maintained at >1 mL/(kg·h), and drugs and CRRT therapy can be used as needed. In addition, attention should also be paid to the fluid loss during ECMO. Fluid can be properly replenished based on central venous pressure, skin elasticity, etc.

The "lung super protective ventilation" strategy should be implemented: Ventilator-related lung injuries should be avoided or reduced as much as possible. It is recommended that the initial tidal volume should be <6 mL/kg. The spontaneous breathing strength should be preserved and the respiratory rate be maintained at 10–20 times/min.

Tubing management: Tubeline should be firmly fixed to avoid detaching and twisting; the tube will shake when the drainage of venous tubeline is open and blood cannot be withdrawn; hemolysis is likely to occur when the negative pressure is too high (above −30 mmHg); pump should be stopped before operation of negative tube system.

Management of pump: The base of centrifugal pump will generate heat and thrombus is likely to develop. When the revolutions are inconsistent with the flow or when hemoglobinurias, etc. appear, it indicates that there may be formation of thrombus. If thrombus develops, abnormal sound of the pump can be heard with a stethoscope.

Infusion management: If possible, fluid infusion and blood transfusion should be carried out after the ECMO. Infusion of those drugs as fat emulsion and Propofol should be avoided.

Infection control: For ECMO, regular air disinfection is required for the ward, and antibiotics should be given for a long term to prevent infection. Attention should be paid on sterile operation and hand hygiene.

7.3.2 Equipment Management During Operation

The water supply, gas supply, and power supply on the tubeline should be checked regularly.

The tubeline should be checked regularly. Power flashlight can be used to check the tubeline and if there is thrombosis on the membrane oxygenation.

The water line of the water temperature tank should be correctly checked.

Whether abnormal sound appears should be observed for the pump head. If there is abnormal sound, it indicates that the pump head is not stably placed in the actuator. The circulation should be stopped and the pump head be removed for replacement.

7.3.3 Management of Common Complications

Equipment failure and pump shutdown: Hand pump should be used to ensure ECMO circulation and safety of the patient. The doctor/perfusionist should be notified and troubleshooting should be carried out. If necessary, instrument should be replaced and the failed one should be sent for repair.

Abnormal function of oxygenator: It is manifested as gas exchange failure, plasma leakage, and thrombosis formation. Hand pump should be used to immediately prefill the new tubeline. The whole set of tubeline should be replaced. The whole team should work together to shorten the shutdown period and ensure safety of the patient.

Air embolism: It is often caused by inappropriate drainage, high negative pressure, cannula displacement, misoperation, etc. The small yellow cap at the venous end/before the membrane should be immediately removed and observation should be strengthened (if there is gas after the membrane). The etiology should be screened. In the case of large volume of gas entry, the circulating gas outlet at the artery end/after the membrane should be stopped. The blood flow should be blocked to prevent the gas from entering the body of the patient. Gas exhaust treatment should be carried out. If necessary, the tubeline should be replaced.

Hemorrhage and hemolysis [1, 8]: Cerebral hemorrhage should be determined by observing the size of the pupil of the patient and other methods. Gastric hemorrhage should be determined by withdrawing the gastric residues and observing the color. Intestinal bleeding should be determined by stool examination. If scleral icterus or jaundice, positive urine occult blood test, coke-colored urine or oliguria, etc., hemolysis or acute kidney injury should be suspected. It is recommended to report to physician for treatment instantly.

7.4 Care of Artificial Liver

Jian Luo

The care of artificial liver is mainly divided into care during the treatment and care in the intermittent phase. Nursing staff should closely observe the disease condition, standardize the operation procedure, and focus on key points and timely handle complications so as to smoothly complete the artificial liver treatment.

7.4.1 Care During the Treatment

Care during the treatment refers to the care during each artificial liver performance. The overall operation procedure can be summarized as follows: Preparation of operator–patient evaluation–machine installation–prefilling–connection of the machine–detaching of the machine record. The key points for care in each step are provided below:

1. Preparation for operators: Protective measures of level III and above should be comprehensively implemented.
2. Patient evaluation: Including clinical status and disease condition of the patient, especially allergic history, blood glucose, coagulation function, oxygen therapy condition, and sedation state. Attention should be paid to the psychological state of conscious patients.
3. Evaluation of catheter state: Routine sterile procedures are recommended during disinfecting the deep venous catheter and wound; draw 2 mL of residual heparin saline from the artery lumen with a 5 mL syringe, push it onto the gauze, and check if there is blood clot; check if 20 mL blood (blood flow is about 200 mL/min) can be withdrawn from the artery lumen with a 20 mL empty syringe in 6 s, push in and repeat once, and then test the blow flow in the artery lumen of the catheter; wash the artery end of the catheter clean with 10 mL of saline; and check the venous end of the catheter by the same method.
4. Installation and prefilling: If possible, closed loop should be used for the treatment tubing and consumables to avoid exposure of the blood and body fluid of

the patient; corresponding instrument, tubing, and other consumables should be selected in accordance with the treatment mode. Medical staff should be familiar with the basic performance of the treatment consumables.

5. Connection of the machine: It is recommended that the initial blood leading speed be ≤50 mL/min to avoid hypotension caused by high velocity; vital signs should be monitored in a timely manner.
6. Parameter adjustment: After extracorporeal circulation becomes stable, treatment parameters and alarm parameters should be adjusted in accordance with the treatment mode; in the early stage, sufficient anticoagulant should be used and the maintenance volume should be adjusted at any time based on the treatment pressure.
7. Detaching of the machine: The liquid plus gravity combined recovery method should be used; the recovery rate should be ≤50 mL/min; after detaching, medical wastes should be disposed and treatment instruments should be cleaned and disinfected in accordance with the prevention and control requirements for SARS-CoV-2 infection.
8. Record: Vital signs of the patient, dosing condition of artificial liver, artificial liver treatment parameters, and remarks of special conditions should be correctly recorded.

7.4.2 Care During the Intermittent Phase

The appearance of hypotension, hemorrhage, coagulation in the catheter in the early stage after treatment and allergic reaction, disequilibrium syndrome, and thrombosis formation in the late stage should be closely observed [9, 10].

Care of artificial liver catheterization: Local condition should be observed and recorded at each shift; catheter-related thrombus should be prevented; professional maintenance of catheter should be carried out every 24 h; access should be fixed properly to avoid twisting and stressing.

Withdrawal of artificial liver catheter: Ultrasound examination of blood vessel should be carried out before withdrawal; after catheter withdrawal, the lower limb at the insertion side should be retaining for 6 h and the patient should stay in bed for 24 h; local trauma should be observed after catheter withdrawal.

7.5 CRRT Care

Jian Luo

7.5.1 Pretreatment Preparations

Preparation of patient: Effective vascular access should be established before CRRT. Generally, central venous catheterization through jugular vein is preferred. If ECMO therapy is planned at the same time, CRRT therapy can be integrated into the ECMO system. The equipment, consumables, and medications for ultrafiltration are prepared ahead.

Catheter evaluation: Disinfecting the deep venous catheter and wound according to general aseptic operation procedure; draw 2 mL of residual heparin saline from the artery lumen with a 5 mL syringe, push it onto the gauze, and check if there is a blood clot; check if 20 mL blood (blood flow is about 200 mL/min) can be withdrawn from the artery lumen with a 20 mL empty syringe in 6 s, push in and repeat once, and then test the blow flow in the artery lumen of the catheter; wash the artery end of the catheter clean with 10 mL of saline; and check the venous end of the catheter by the same method.

7.5.2 Care During Treatment

Maintenance of vascular access: Before accessing the catheter, the state of the catheter should be evaluated. During use, tubing should be properly fixed to avoid twisting and stressing.

The machine control system should be adjusted. The blood flow velocity in the beginning of dialysis should be slow (50 mL/min), then can be gradually increased, and reach 200 mL/min in about 15 min. After the blood flow becomes stable, alarm thresholds should be set.

The consciousness of patients and changes in vital signs should be closely monitored and the in- and output of fluid should be correctly calculated; the coagulation condition of extracorporeal circulation should be closely observed and alarms should be effectively handled to ensure smooth operation of the machine; blood gas should be monitored and analyzed every 4 h; and acid–base equilibrium of electrolytes in the internal environment should be evaluated.

The aseptic operation principle should be strictly applied and hand hygiene should be strictly implemented. The aseptic operation principle should be strictly followed for the configuration of substitution fluid. Substitution fluid should be prepared upon use, with clear label.

Observation of common complications: (1) hypotension: it is related to too much and rapid ultrafiltration dehydration, insufficient blood volume, cardiogenic shock, inhibition of acetate to myocardium, or allergy. It may be accompanied by nausea, vomiting, pale complexion, chest tightness, sweating, and even transient loss of consciousness. (2) Disequilibrium syndrome: It is likely to occur when patients have severe azotemia with high content of urea and is manifested as headache, nausea and vomiting, hypertension, convulsion, and coma for severe patients. (3) Pyrogenic reaction: Often occurs 1 h after the beginning of dialysis. It is caused by endotoxin entering the body and manifested as chill followed by fever. (4) Hemorrhage: It is often caused by the application of heparin, platelet dysfunction, and hypertension. It is often manifested as nasal bleeding, gum bleeding, gastrointestinal hemorrhage, intracranial haemorrhage, etc.

Record: Arterial pressure, variceal pressure, transmembrane pressure, blood flow rate, rate of substitution fluid, ultrafiltration volume, and other indicators should be recorded hourly.

7.5.3 Care Posttreatment

Blood routine, liver and kidney function, and coagulation function of the patient should be monitored.

Maintenance of indwelling catheter: Indwelling catheter should be properly fixed and flushed and sealed regularly. Catheter puncture point should be covered with sterile dressing, and dressing change should be carried out regularly. Upon dressing change, attention should be paid to the skin around the opening of the catheter for redness, swelling, warmness, tenderness, and blood and fluid leakage.

Equipment in continuous operation should be wiped and disinfected every 24 h, and consumables and waste liquid should be disposed in accordance with the hospital's requirements for prevention of infection.

7.6 Care of PICC, CVC, and Medium-Long Catheter

Jian Luo

7.6.1 Preparation Before Catheterization

Level III protection should be provided for operators. Absolute contraindications should be avoided. During catheterization, technical specification for sterile operation should be strictly followed and needle stick injuries should be prevented.

7.6.2 Care During Use [10]

Catheter should be flushed with 20 mL of saline by impulsion and positive pressure before usage. Flushing and dosing with syringe less than 10 mL should be avoided. Violent flushing should be avoided to prevent damaging the catheter.

The sterile operation procedure should be strictly followed. Dressing and the positive pressure joint should be replaced every 7 days. Dressing change should be carried out timely in case of edge curling, looseness, and sweating under the sticking film dressing. Positive pressure joint should be replaced immediately after catheter flushing after blood infusion, blood drawing, and infusion of such high-viscosity drugs as fat emulsion.

The responsible nurse should observe the condition of the catheter at each shift to avoid detaching of the catheter, redness, swelling, warmness, tenderness, leakage, etc. around the needle eye, and discover and solve these problems as early as possible.

Blood pressure measurement at the limb of the catheter side should be avoided. Patients should be instructed to carry out functional exercise every day to avoid thrombus.

Care of post-catheter withdrawal: The insertion site should be pressed for 10 min after catheter withdrawal, and the wound be locally sealed with sealing gauze and transparent film dressing for 48 h. As the puncture hole at the vascular access is big, movement stretching should be prevented to prevent air from entering or bleeding of the wound.

Preventive measures for implementing unplanned catheter withdrawal. Adverse safety events arising from withdrawing and environmental contamination by aerosol during withdrawal should be avoided.

"Patient health questionnaire PHQ-9 risk evaluation" should be carried out when the patients are admitted to the hospital. High-risk patients should be screened and mental care be provided for patients. Take care of patients' psychological changes.

References

1. Nursing standard for patients with severe and critical COVID-19; General Office of National Health Commission.
2. Zhong N, Hao Q, Jie L, et al. Consensus on management of nasal high-flow oxygen therapy in patients with COVID-19 [J/OL]. Chin J Respir Crit Care Med. 1–7 [2020-03-25]. http://kns.cnki.net/kcms/detail/51.1631.r.20200218.1536.002.html.
3. WHO. Clinical management of severe acute respiratory infection when novel coronavirus (2019-nCoV) infection is suspected: interim guidance.
4. Zhang W, Pan C, Song Q. We should pay close attention to some issues in the process of respiratory therapy of COVID-19 [J/OL]. Med J Chin People's Liber Army. 1–6 [2020-03-25]. http://kns.cnki.net/kcms/detail/11.1056.r.20200226.1950.004.html.
5. Xu K, Cai H, Shen Y, et al. Management of corona virus disease-19 (COVID-19): the Zhejiang experience [J/OL]. J Zhejiang Univ (Med Sci). 1–12 [2020-03-25]. http://kns.cnki.net/kcms/detail/33.1248.R.20200222.1417.002.html.
6. Ge H, Dai B, Xu P, et al. Consensus on control of ventilator infection of patients with COVID-19 [J/OL]. Chin J Respir Crit Care Med. 1–4 [2020-03-25]. http://kns.cnki.net/kcms/detail/51.1631.R.20200210.2248.002.html.
7. Ren W, Shen L, Zhao M, et al. Nursing challenge of most critically ill COVID-19 patients and its strategies: a 12-case study [J/OL]. J Nurs (China). 1–4 [2020-03-25]. http://kns.cnki.net/kcms/detail/44.1631.R.20200323.1217.012.html.
8. Liu X, Li Y, Cai L, et al. Nursing care of critically ill patients treated with extracorporeal membrane oxygenation combined with continuous renal replacement therapy [J]. Nurs Integr Tradit Chin West Med. 2020;6(01):109–12.
9. Liver Failure and Artificial Liver Group, Branch of Infectious Diseases, Chinese Medical Association. Guideline for non-bioartificial liver support systems in treatment of liver failure: 2016 update [J]. Chin J Clin Infect Dis. 2016;9(2):97–103. (in Chinese)
10. Sun H, Chen L, Guo C, et al. Expert consensus on venous catheter maintenance [J]. Chin J Nurs. 2019;54(09):1334–42.

Guidelines and Guidance 8

Fanjun Cheng and Jianchu Zhang

Contents

8.1 Guidance on Clinical Practice

Fanjun Cheng

8.1.1 Treatment Protocol for Severe and Critical COVID-19 Patients: Experiences from Wuhan Union Hospital

Note: This section is reprinted with permission from: Yong Gao, et al. Treatment protocol for severe and critical COVID-19 patients: Experiences from Wuhan Union Hospital. Current Medical Science (ISSN: 2096-5230), 2020, Springer. Accepted article.

The corresponding author of Sect. 8.1 is Fanjun Cheng, Email: chengfanjun001@sina.com
The corresponding author of Sect. 8.2 is Jianchu Zhang, Email: zsn0928@163.com

F. Cheng (✉)
Department of Internal Medicine, Union Hospital, Tongji Medical College of Huazhong University of Science and Technology, Wuhan, China

J. Zhang
Department of Respiratory and Critical Care Medicine, Union Hospital, Tongji Medical College, Huazhong University of Science and Technology, Wuhan, China

F. Cheng, Y. Zhang (eds.), *The Clinical Diagnosis and Treatment for New Coronavirus Pneumonia*, https://doi.org/10.1007/978-981-15-5975-4_8

Abstract
In late December 2019, a newly emerging infectious disease, COVID-19, was identified in Wuhan, China. COVID-19 spread rapidly to the entire country of China with a mortality rate of 2–4%. The West Campus of Wuhan Union Hospital, the designated hospital for admitting and treating the severe and critical COVID-19 cases, has been treating a large number of patients with great success. To standardize and share the treatment protocol for severe and critical cases, Wuhan Union Hospital has established a working group and formulated an operational guideline, including monitoring, early warning indicators, and several treatment principles for severe and critical cases.

Keywords
2019-nCoV, COVID-19, Pneumonia, Treatment guidelines

Background

An ongoing outbreak of pneumonia caused by the 2019 novel coronavirus (2019-nCoV, now formally named SARS-CoV-2 by the International Committee on Taxonomy of Viruses, ICTV) has been recently identified as a newly emerging infectious disease. 2019-nCov is highly contagious, and it has a significant morbidity and 2–4% mortality rate. 2019-nCoV disease (named COVID-19 by the WHO) was first identified in Wuhan in late December 2019. It subsequently spread rapidly to the whole country and then to multiple countries and almost all over the world. The 2019-nCoV virus belongs to a novel type of β genus coronavirus that shares 79.5% sequence with severe acute respiratory syndrome-related coronaviruses (SARS-CoV). It mainly, but not exclusively, attacks the human respiratory system in severe and critical cases. Among the infected patients, about 14% were severe and 5% were critically ill with cellular immune deficiency, coagulation activation, cytokine storm, myocardia injury, and hepatic and kidney injury. According to minimally invasive autopsies, we learned that the lungs from COVID-19 patients manifest significant pathological changes and the injury also involves damage to the heart, vessels, liver, kidney, and other organs.

Chinese health institutions enacted immediate measures to control the disease, including isolation of suspected people, close monitoring of contacts, collection of epidemiological and clinical data, and development of diagnostic and treatment guidelines. The West Campus of Wuhan Union Hospital, as one of the three designated hospitals appointed by the National Health Commission of China for admitting and treating the severe and critical COVID-19 cases, has recruited the largest number of these patients.

Until March 20, 2020, 1617 patients were diagnosed with severe and critical types of COVID-19 disease. After treatment, 1069 patients were cured and discharged, and 147 died. Currently, there are still 401 patients under treatment. The high cure rate and control from spreading confirms the effectiveness of our management and treatment protocol. Currently, the pandemic in other countries is still serious, which has prompted international concern about the global public health impact. To standardize and share the treatment protocol of severe and critical cases, Wuhan Union Hospital has established a working group and formulated the following operational recommendations for treating severe and critical patients. The protocol is based on the Chinese guideline (V7.0) and previous experiences accumulated from the isolation ward over the past 2 months.

8.1.1.1 Establishment of Baseline Disease Data on Admission

8.1.1.1.1 History Collection

Upon admission, full clinical data from the patients should be accurately collected. This serves as a starting point for observation and disease control. The data to be obtained include epidemiological history, clinical manifestations, as well as the diagnosis and treatment history from other medical institutions. The severe and critical patients should be diagnosed according to the guidelines of the National Health Commission of China (V7.0). All of the data should be collected during treatment, and a flowchart should be established to depict and predict disease evolution.

8.1.1.1.2 Auxiliary Examinations

On admission, patients are required to complete the following tests:

1. Complete blood count, lymphocyte subsets
2. C-reactive protein (CRP), erythrocyte sedimentation rate (ESR), procalcitonin (PCT), and inflammatory cytokines (including IL-6, IL-10, and TNF-α)
3. Hepatic and renal functions and electrolytes
4. Disseminated intravascular coagulation (DIC) screening (including coagulation function and D-dimer)
5. Blood gas analysis
6. Chest X-ray or CT scan
7. Others: Troponin, cardiac enzymes, B-type natriuretic peptide, lactate dehydrogenase (LDH), creatine kinase, and myoglobin

It is recommended that the severe patients should be monitored with these accessory laboratory tests every 3 days, and critically ill patients daily except for radiographic images. The evolution curve can be generated through a data management program.

8.1.1.1.3 Detection of Pathogens

1. 2019-nCoV detection: 2019-nCoV nucleic acid can be detected with nasopharyngeal swabs, sputum, lower respiratory tract secretions, blood, feces, and other specimens utilizing RT-PCR or NGS methods. The accuracy of RNA 2019-nCoV detection is as follows: Alveolar lavage fluid > sputum > nasal swab > throat swab. 2019-nCoV-specific IgM becomes detectable via serological tests at 3–5 days post-onset, and an IgG-positive test indicates previous infection and

convalescence. The combined detection of viral RNA and serology in COVID-19 patients can improve the sensitivity and specificity of diagnosis.
2. Secondary bacterial and fungal pathogenic tests: Severe and critical patients with COVID-19 are susceptible to bacterial and fungal infections, and clinical microbiological test should be monitored.
3. Metagenomic sequencing (mNGS): mNGS has obvious advantages of comprehensive detection, high accuracy, high sensitivity, and fast identification over RT-PCR, which significantly improves not only the detection efficiency of COVID-19, but also co-infection and secondary infection of severe and critical COVID-19 patients.
4. Sampling, transportation, and testing involving pathogenic inspections must meet biosafety requirements.

8.1.1.1.4 Comorbidities and Complications Monitoring

1. Most of the patients with the severe and critical type of COVID-19 are relatively elders and generally have a variety of comorbidities. These pathophysiological factors have a great impact on the diagnosis, treatment, and prognosis of COVID-19, which should be noted and monitored.
2. 2019-nCoV affects multiple organs other than the respiratory system, including cardiovascular, gastrointestinal, blood, and immunity, and the appropriate tests should be carried out as needed.
3. No specific drugs have yet been produced. Although several types of clinically therapeutic drugs have been tested, the interactions between drugs and drug side effects are not clear and should be taken into consideration. The clinical pharmacy-related tests are required when necessary.

8.1.1.2 Early Clinical Warning Signs of Severe and Critical Cases

Previous experiences have revealed that some COVID-19 cases can progress and deteriorate to moderate, severe, or critical ones in a short period of time. The cases with the following indicators are likely to deteriorate to severe or critical status. Early warning and treatment will be of great importance to reduce mortality.

1. The age of the patient has an independent prognosis factor, and the 2019-nCoV-infected patients with the age of ≥65 years old or ≥75 years old are separately prone to the severe or critical type.
2. The progressive decline of peripheral blood lymphocytes indicates the deterioration of the disease.
3. Abnormality in DIC screening tests suggests the deterioration of the disease.
4. Lung lesions >50% in size or involving the inner band suggest the progression of the disease.
5. Patients with serious underlying diseases (including structural lung disease, coronary heart disease, critical hypertension, rheumatic immune disease, neoplastic disease, or other infectious diseases), immunosuppressive treatment, organ transplantation, blood purification, and chemotherapy have a poor prognostic outcome.

8.1.1.3 Principles for Treating the Severe and Critical Patients

1. Basic treatment
   (a) Bed rest with strong nutritional support.
   (b) Maintain water, electrolyte, and acid–base balance.
   (c) Energy mixture, ATP, or CoA can be used for anti-hypoxia treatment.
   (d) Underlying diseases should be treated.
   (e) Measures should be taken to prevent secondary infection.
   (f) Prevent and treat complications, including cardiac injury, cardiogenic shock, myocarditis, venous thrombosis (VTE), DIC, ventilator-induced dysfunctions, and multifunctional organ failure.
   (g) Cytokine storm treatment
2. Antiviral therapy

   The following antiviral drugs are recommended within 10 days of COVID-19 onset, but at best, no more than two drugs in combination: *ribavirin* (500 mg for adults, twice or three times via intravenous injection daily, administered no longer than 10 days), *lopinavir/ritonavir* (used to be recommended by Chinese guidelines, but it was recently reported that no benefit was observed with lopinavir/ritonavir treatment beyond standard care in a randomized, controlled, open-label trial), *chloroquine phosphate* (500 mg for 7 days for adults aged 18–65 with body weight over 50 kg; 500 mg for days 1 and 2, and 500 mg for days 3–7 for adults with body weight below 50 kg), *hydroxychloroquine* (found to be more potent than chloroquine at inhibiting 2019-nCoV in vitro), and *Arbidol* (200 mg tid for adults, no longer than 10 days). Some medicine under clinical trial can also be tried if the above antiviral treatments fail to work. Be aware of adverse reactions, contraindications (e.g., chloroquine cannot be used for patients with heart diseases), and interactions of the abovementioned drugs. If an intolerable toxic side effect occurs, the respective drug should be discontinued.
3. Oxygen Therapy and Respiratory Support
   (A) **High-flow nasal-catheter oxygenation (HFNC)** is suitable for patients with hypoxemia and oxygenation index (PaO_2/FiO_2) of 200–300 mmHg. During the implementation of HFNC treatment, the symptoms and signs of the patients should be closely monitored and evaluated every 20–30 min. The following conditions indicate failure of HFNC treatment, and alternative respiratory support therapy should be added:
      (a) Hypoxemia not able to correct ($SpO_2 < 93\%$)
      (b) Tachypnea (RR $\geq$ 35 beats/min)
      (c) Significantly difficult to inspirates
   (B) **Noninvasive ventilator (NIV)** is suitable for patients with hypoxemia and PaO_2/FiO_2 of 150–200 mmHg. During the implementation of NIV treatment, the symptoms and signs of the patients should be closely monitored and evaluated every 20–30 min. The following situations indicate failure of NIV treatment, and alternative respiratory support therapy should be considered in time:
      (a) Hypoxemia not able to correct ($SpO_2 < 93\%$)
      (b) Tachypnea (RR $\geq$ 35 beats/min)

   (c) Excessive tidal volume
   (d) Excessive negative inspiratory pressure
   (e) Unstable circulation and abnormal tissue perfusion

(C) **Invasive mechanical ventilation (IMV)** is suitable for patients with hypoxemia and PaO_2/FiO_2 < 150 mmHg. Based on lung protective ventilation strategy, patients with hypoxemia and PaO_2/FiO_2 < 150 mmHg require repeated monitoring of the lung recruitment maneuver potential. Use the PEEP strategy to restore the lung potential and closely observe the oxygenation index, pressure of carbon dioxide, right heart enlargement, and pulmonary barotrauma. Prone position ventilation is recommended. Patients who have reached the following conditions can withdraw mechanical ventilation: PaO_2/FiO_2 maintains >200 mmHg, the primary disease is improved, the patient gains consciousness, and the patient is dynamically stable.

(D) **Extracorporeal membrane oxygenation (ECMO)**

Indications of ECMO therapy:

   (a) PaO_2/FiO_2 < 50 mmHg for more than 3 h
   (b) PaO_2/FiO_2 < 80 mmHg for more than 6 h
   (c) FiO_2 1.0, PaO_2/FiO_2 < 100 mmHg
   (d) Arterial blood pH < 7.25 and $PaCO_2$ > 60 mmHg more than 6 h, or related complications caused by carbon dioxide retention: severe internal environment disorder and right heart failure
   (e) When the respiratory rate >35 per min, the arterial blood pH < 7.2, and the airway plateau pressure >30 cm H_2O
   (f) Combined with cardiogenic shock or cardiac arrest

Contraindications of ECMO therapy: Combined with irreversible primary diseases, contraindication for anticoagulation, ventilation for more than 7 days under a higher mechanical ventilation setting (FiO_2 > 0.9, airway plateau pressure >30 cm H_2O), age >70 years old, the use of immunosuppression, and the presence of peripheral vascular anatomical malformations or vascular lesions.

4. Rational use of antibiotics
   (a) Avoid blind or inappropriate use of antibiotics if there is no clear evidence of bacterial infection.
   (b) For severe and critical cases with a course of disease ≥7 days, surveillance of pathogens related to secondary bacterial or fungal infection should be effectively carried out.
   (c) Bacterial infection should be suspected and confirmed according to body temperature, white blood cell count (WBC), neutrophil percentage, pulmonary imaging, oxygenation function, and pathogen examination. The third-generation cephalosporin/enzyme inhibitor complex can be empirically used.
   (d) When septic shock occurs in severe and critically ill patients, carbapenem drugs can be used instead. If enterococcal and staphylococcal infections are suspected, glycopeptide antibiotics (vancomycin) can be added for empirical treatment.

(e) Be especially cautious to catheter-related infections. Empirical antibiotic treatment should cover methicillin-resistant staphylococci with the use of glycopeptide drugs (vancomycin).

(f) Some patients often have secondary aspergillosis infection in the later stages of critical illness. Voriconazole can be used, but the combination of two antifungal drugs is not recommended.

5. Prophylactic anticoagulant therapy

(a) Severe and critically ill COVID-19 patients have a higher risk for DIC and VTE. Coagulation and bleeding should be closely monitored during treatment. Unless there is significant bleeding or a coagulation disease, low-molecular-weight heparin is recommended for the vast majority of critically ill patients.

(b) When DIC occurs and there is no significant hyperfibrinolysis, a therapeutic dose of low-molecular-weight heparin can be added, but with simultaneous replacement therapy such as platelet transfusion, and/or supplemented with fresh plasma to replenish coagulation factors; hematologists should be invited for consultation as soon as possible.

(c) The risk of VTE in severe and critically ill patients should be regularly assessed according to the Caprini Risk Assessment Model: when the score >3, medication and physical prophylaxis are recommended. Encourage patients to exercise at an early stage and invite a vascular surgeon to consult when VTE is suspected.

6. Convalescent plasma treatment

The 2019-nCoV-specific antibodies in the plasma of COVID-19 convalescent patients have a certain therapeutic effect on COVID-19 patients via reducing 2019-nCoV viral copy numbers. Convalescent plasma treatment can be used for severe patients above 18 years of age and only for the certain critical patients with mechanical ventilation ≤48 h and heart, liver, and kidney function still being in a compensatory state.

7. IL-6 monoclonal antibody treatment

Cytokine release syndrome (CRS), which is closely associated with the increased level of IL-6, is an important cause of death in critically ill patients with COVID-19. It is speculated that the IL-6 monoclonal antibody (Tocilizumab) can inhibit the intensity of the cytokine storm and play a certain therapeutic role. IL-6 monoclonal antibody therapy is suitable for severe patients >18 years of age without severe comorbidities and contraindicated for patients with active infections, such as tuberculosis.

8. Glucocorticoid treatment

Currently, there is no evidence to support that the medical use of glucocorticoids improves the prognosis of severe COVID-19 patients. However, patients with progressive deterioration of oxygenation indicators, rapid progress in imaging, excessive activation of the body's inflammatory response, and without contraindications can use conventional doses of glucocorticoids in a short period of time (3–5 days).

9. Other recommended treatments

   There is no clinical evidence to support the application of drugs such as human immunoglobulin, thymosin, and intestinal microecological regulators to improve the prognosis of severe COVID-19 patients. They are recommended as supplemental therapeutic measures.
10. Traditional Chinese Medicine

    COVID-19 belongs to the category of traditional Chinese medicine plagues. Dialectical treatment based on factors, such as seasonal and geographical aspects, has played an important role in the prevention and control of the COVID-19 epidemic in China from 2019 to 2020. According to the different local climate characteristic and individual state of illness and physical conditions, Chinese medicine prescriptions and Western medicines can be used alone or in combination.

Summary

2019-nCoV is a recently identified novel pathogen with great contagiousness and susceptibility among the human population. Based on the guidelines of the diagnosis and treatment of COVID-19, comprehensive supportive treatment is still the major treatment procedure before the development of specific antiviral drugs and effective vaccines.

Experts in the working group:

- **HaiboQiu**, Zhongda hospital of Southeast University, Nanjing.
- **Zhenning Wang**, The First Affiliated Hospital of China Medical University, Shenyang.
- **Zhengliang Zhang**, The Second Affiliated Hospital of Xi'an Jiaotong University, Xi'an.
- **Zhaoxin Qian**, Xiangya Hospital of Zhongnan University, Changsha.
- **Shihuan Yu**, The First Affiliated Hospital of Harbin Medical University, Harbin.
- **Yifeng Luo**, The First Affiliated Hospital of Sun Yat-sen University, Guangzhou.
- **Zhuang Liu**, Beijing Friendship Hospital of Capital Medical University, Beijing.
- **Ming Jia,** Beijing Anzhen Hospital of Capital Medical University, Beijing.
- **Liming Zhang**, Beijing Chaoyang Hospital of Capital Medical University, Beijing.
- And my colleagues **Yong Gao, Yadan Wang, Hongbo Wang, Jianchu Zhang, Shu Zhou, Weici Wang, Yu Zhang, Yang Jin, Yong Zhang, Yong Liu, Zihua Zhou, Ying Su, Huiqing Li, WeiminXiao, Kai Huang, Ping He, Gang Li, Zhaohui Fu, Shi Liu, Nengxing Lin**, et al. from Union Hospital, Tongji Medical College, Huazhong University of Science and Technology, Wuhan. We appreciate all of the physicians and nurses who share their valuable experiences and for their hard work in treating COVID-19 patients, and for those who have contributed to translating and proofreading the manuscript.

8.2 Modular Medical Orders

Jianchu Zhang

8.2.1 Example Medical Order for Mild Patient with COVID-19

Medical Order for Diagnosis and Treatment

- Air isolation, body temperature measurement (q4h), monitoring the oxygen saturation (q6d), heart rate/blood pressure checking (q6h)

  Medical Order for Accessory Tests

- Nucleic acid testing for SARS-CoV-2
- Routine blood test, biochemical test, routine urine test, routine stool test+OB, CPR, respiratory viral test
- ECG, CT of the lung

  Medical Prescriptions

- Arbidol tablets 200 mg tid
- or Favipiravir tablets D1 1600 mg bid; then change to 600 mg bid

8.2.2 Example Medical Order for Moderate Patient with COVID-19

Medical Order for Diagnosis and Treatment

- Air isolation, body temperature measurement (q4h), monitoring of oxygen saturation (q6h), heart rate/blood pressure test (q6h)

  Medical Order for accessory tests

- Nucleic acid testing for SARS-CoV-2
- Routine blood test, biochemical test, routine urine test, routine stool test+OB, coagulation function+D-dimer, CPR, ESR, PCT, myocardial enzyme+quantitative test of serum cardiac troponin T, respiratory tract virus test, blood/sputum culture (recheck every 3–5 days)
- B-ultrasonic examination of deep veins of both lower limbs, ultrasonic examination of the heart, CT of the lung, EKG

Medical Prescriptions

- Arbidol tablets 200 mg tid
- or Lopinavir and ritonavir tablets 400/100 mg q12h
- or Favipiravir tablets: D1 1600 mg bid; then change to 600 mg bid
- Acetylcysteine tablets 600 mg, dissolve and take after meal bid

8.2.3 Example Medical Order for Severe Patient with COVID-19

Medical Order for Diagnosis and Treatment

- Air isolation, ECG monitoring, monitoring of oxygen saturation/body temperature, heart rate q4h, oxygen therapy support (oxygen supply by nasal cannula, oxygen supply by mask, HFNC, NIV)

Medical Order for Accessory Tests

- Nucleic acid testing for SARS-CoV-2
- Routine blood test, biochemical test, routine urine test, routine stool test+PB, coagulation function+D-dimer, BNP, blood gas analysis+lactic acid, ASO+RF+CPR, ESR, PCT, thyroid function, ferritin, myocardial enzyme+quantitative test of serum cardiac troponin T, respiratory tract virus test, blood/sputum culture, immunoglobulin+complement, T-lymphocyte subsets, cytokine, G/GM test (recheck every 2–3 days)
- B-ultrasonic examination of deep veins of both lower limbs, ultrasonic examination of the heart, CT of the lung, EKG

Medical Prescriptions

- Arbidol tablets 200 mg tid
- Lopinavir and ritonavir tablets 400/100 mg q12h
- α-Interferon (add 5,000,000 IU into 2 mL of saline for aerosol inhalation, bid)
- NS100ML+Methylprednisolone 40 mg iv gtt qd (when necessary)
- NS100ML+Pantoprazole for injection 40 mg qd (when hormone is used)
- Caltrate D, one tablet qd
- Low-molecular-weight heparin sodium (Clexane) 4000 U ih qd or bid (when there is no obvious anticoagulant contraindications)
- NS100ML+Ambroxol 30 mg iv gtt bid or acetylcysteine tablets 600 mg dissolve and take after meal bid

8.2.4 Example Medical Orders for Critical Patient with COVID-19

Medical Order for Diagnosis and Treatment

- Air isolation, ECG monitoring, monitoring of oxygen saturation/heart rate/blood pressure q1h, body temperature monitoring q4h, prevention and care of high risk pressure sore, oral care, nasal feeding, blood glucose monitoring q6h, 24-h intake and output volume, breathing support (HFNC, NIV, invasive positive pressure ventilation, ECMO)

Medical Order for Accessory Tests

- Nucleic acid testing for SARS-CoV-2
- Routine blood test qd, biochemical test qd, routine urine test, routine stool test+OB, coagulation function+D-dimer qd, blood gas analysis+lactic acid bid, BNP qd, ASO+RF+CPR qd, ESR, PCT qd, thyroid function, ferritin, myocardial enzyme+quantitative test of serum cardiac troponin T qd, respiratory tract virus test, blood culture, immunoglobulin+complement, T-lymphocyte subsets, cytokine, G/GM test
- EKG, B-ultrasonic examination of deep veins of both lower limbs, ultrasonic examination of the heart, CT of the lung, X-ray monitoring of chest at bedside (qd)

Medical Prescriptions

- Arbidol tablets 200 mg tid
- Lopinavir and ritonavir tablets two tablets q12h
- α-Interferon (add 5,000,000 IU into 2 mL of saline for aerosol inhalation, bid)
- NS100ML+Methylprednisolone 40 mg iv gtt q12h, reduce 3 days later in accordance with the actual condition (when necessary)
- NS100ML+Pantoprazole for injection 40 mg qd (when hormone is used)
- Caltrate D, one tablet qd
- Immunoglobulin for injection 0.4 g/kg (15–20 g/day) iv gtt qd
- Empiric antibiotic therapy
- Immunoglobulin for injection 20 g iv gtt qd
- Thymosin for injection 1.6 mg iv biw
- Low-molecular-weight heparin sodium (Clexane) 4000 U ih qd or bid (when there is no obvious anticoagulant contraindications)
- Human serum albumin 10 g iv gtt qd (albumin <30 g/L)
- NS100ML+Ambroxol 30 mg iv gtt bid or acetylcysteine tablets 600 mg bid
- Enteral nutritional suspension: Supportan or Fresubin, or Nutrison Fiber or Peptison, 20–30 kcal/kg

8.3 Diagnosis and Treatment Protocol for Novel Coronavirus Pneumonia (Trial Version 7)

Released by National Health Commission & State Administration of Traditional Chinese Medicine on March 3, 2020.

Links site: http://shliangshi.com/newsshow_825.html

Or scan QR code below:

Postscript

Fanjun Cheng and Yu Zhang

The English version of *The Clinical Diagnosis and Treatment for New Coronavirus Pneumonia* is about to be printed after intensive writing and translation. At this point, the spread of COVID-19 is mostly under control. The center of the epidemic, Wuhan, a metropolis located in the hinterland of China, has been officially reopened for 76 days after the city lockdown, and the medical teams which came from different provinces of China have completed their mission and returned. The epidemic prevention and control in Wuhan by now have focused on the physical rehabilitation of patients, management of asymptomatic infected people, prevention of epidemic recurrence, and orderly recovery of urban function and economic operation. However, the turning point for the epidemic has not yet come worldwide. More than 160 countries and regions have been suffering from COVID-19, with more than 1.6 million confirmed cases, and people in these countries and regions need urgent support and reinforcement. We feel sympathy for those in the same situation as we experienced in Wuhan and want to aid as many people as possible.

The book began at the most difficult time of COVID-19 prevention and control in China. In the face of the new fulminating infectious disease caused by a new pathogen, medical staff and scientific researchers from Wuhan Union Hospital of China combined with clinicians from 21 national medical teams have accumulated experience during the exploration. Since we became more familiar with the disease, an epidemic prevention and control system along with diagnosis and treatment practice with Chinese characteristics was rapidly established. The predecessor of this book is an internal publication which was issued on January 8, 2020, by Wuhan Union Hospital, a hospital for severe and critical disease treatment designated by the Chinese government. From February 19, this publication was printed and distributed nationwide as an attachment by the Joint Prevention and Control Mechanism of the State Council—the highest command authority for COVID-19 prevention and control in China, and has played a key role in the significant stage victory of COVID-19 prevention and control. As the COVID-19 prevention and control continue to advance, Chinese doctors and scientists are more knowledgeable about the

F. Cheng, Y. Zhang (eds.), *The Clinical Diagnosis and Treatment for New Coronavirus Pneumonia*, https://doi.org/10.1007/978-981-15-5975-4

occurrence, development, diagnosis, treatment, and control of the disease. However, there may be some mistakes and deficiencies in the book since there is still a long way to go to get a full and systematic understanding of COVID-19. We will continue to follow up on COVID-19 research, such as clinical reports, clinical studies, experimental studies, and epidemiological investigation results. The above findings will be used in updating and revising the book so as to ensure it covers the latest developments of the COVID-19 pandemic.

Wuhan, China
April 19, 2020

Fanjun Cheng
Yu Zhang

MIX
Papier aus verantwortungsvollen Quellen
Paper from responsible sources
FSC® C105338

If you have any concerns about our products,
you can contact us on
ProductSafety@springernature.com

In case Publisher is established outside the EU,
the EU authorized representative is:
Springer Nature Customer Service Center GmbH
Europaplatz 3, 69115 Heidelberg, Germany

Printed by Libri Plureos GmbH
in Hamburg, Germany